365 Days to Embracing Forbidden Emotions

A Daily Guide to Peace and Fulfillment

JEBWizard Publishing
Books with Character

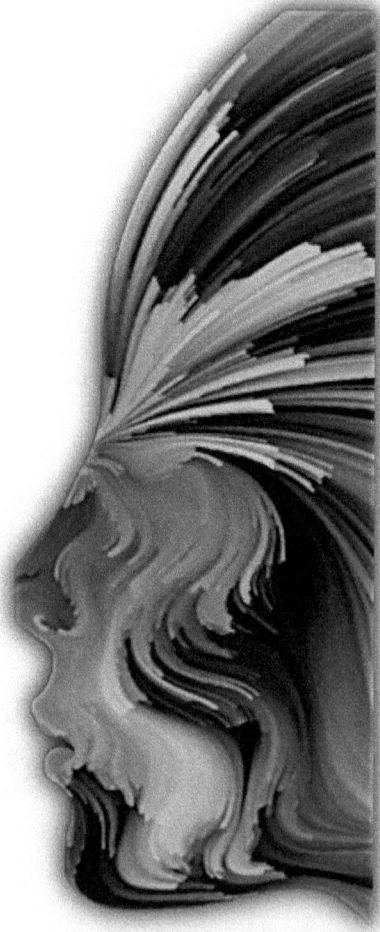

365 Days to Embracing Forbidden Emotions
A Daily Guide to Peace and Fulfillment

By Marti Murphy and Bailey Samples

JEBWizard Publishing
Books with Character

Copyright

Printed in the United States of America by Ingramspark

First Printing, December 2020

ISBN 978-1-7335264-1-8 (Print)

ISBN 978-1-7343553-1-4 (eBook)

JEBWizard Publishing37 Park Forest RD, Cranston, RI 02920

www.jebwizardpublishing.com

Dedication

Dedicated to all who feel they have lost their way in the ego's world of emotional suppression and spiritual materialism.

May this help you heal through feeling fully and freely.

May this help you find the light within you that guides you through this life and brings you back home to your most authentic self.

JEBWizard Publishing
Books with Character

Table of Contents

Introduction

This book is both a supplemental guide to the first book, Forbidden Emotions - The Key to Healing, and a standalone daily guide to help you make micro-changes that lead to profound shifts in your life. Some concepts repeat throughout the book intentionally. The purpose is to help you practice these concepts frequently, so you embody them and see lasting results.

In this book, the word ego, and the terms inner bully and bully in your brain are interchangeable. The bully in your brain is a term I've used to call the ego, because in my experience in my own life and with clients, that's how it feels.

When the ego is yammering away incessantly with all of its shoulds, have to's, and the fear and anxiety it promotes within you, it can feel like a school yard bully that's beating you up emotionally and ultimately physically because of the stress load you carry.

As you learn to recognize this inner bully (the ego) running your show, you can interrupt it with tapping and/or the simple, yet powerful, mental noting. Over time, these interruptions have a profound and healing impact on your wellbeing.

The **_THOUGHT FOR THE DAY_** is usually presented in 'What if' statements because the brain is more open to suggestions that start with the bridging words, 'What if?' This is because 'What if' carries less resistance which allows you to use the suggestions in a helpful way.

God, The Universe, the authentic self, the higher self, force of good are all used interchangeably. Whatever you need to call a spiritual force or wiser part of yourself that guides you through this life, as you open to it and deepen this connection.

If you're looking to go deeper into this work you may find the first book, Forbidden Emotions - The Key to Healing helpful as it has foundational concepts that can assist you in a profound way.

Here's to embracing your unique journey,

Marti Murphy and Bailey Samples

January

January 1

"Use pain as a stepping-stone, not a campground." Alan Cohen

When I hear this quote, I might think, "of course, I don't want to stay stuck in pain," yet I can feel incapable of moving beyond it, when feeling it feels forbidden. So what do I do when my mind conflicts with my heart?

I can tap through the pain. I can acknowledge, honor, and go deeper into the pain, so I can release it from my body, my mind and ultimately my spirit.

What does going into the pain mean? It means instead of telling myself I shouldn't feel whatever I'm feeling, I actually do the opposite. I give the pain my full attention. I allow it to open up within me without the should nots and shoulds I place on myself. The should nots and shoulds only hold the pain in place, indefinitely, which doesn't allow me to move beyond it. The culture I live in can tell me to just "let it go," but how do I do this? I do it by honoring the truth of my pain and allowing it to move through me using tapping. With tapping supporting me I can give the pain it's full, unadulterated expression, which is a highly effective way to find relief.

What you find on the other side of the pain is liberation, freedom, peace of mind and peace within the pain, because you are no longer impeding the flow of pain. You are allowing its full expression and your gift is emotional, mental, physical, and spiritual freedom.

THOUGHT FOR THE DAY: *As I allow myself to tap through the fullness of my pain and find freedom.*

January 2

"Feelings are like waves. You cannot stop them from coming but you can decide which ones to surf." Unknown

---

I have times in my life, maybe more than I care to admit, where my emotions run me. I'm unable to decide as to which feelings I surf.

Feelings have a way of just showing up on my doorstep. Often, I open the door before ever looking through the window or asking who's there, to discover which ones are knocking at my door.

So what can I do? I can start with awareness. When I notice my emotions are running me, what if I just accomplished the first step...I noticed? I learn my emotions have a grip on me. This is a huge accomplishment as I learn to acknowledge this big win. Awareness is the first step in effecting any real changes in my life.

Through my awareness, I can now tap to interrupt and thus slow the momentum of the emotions. When tapping, my feelings may intensify, at first, but that's actually a good things. It's good, because the intensity is letting me know I've targeted a deeper level of the emotions. As I keep tapping, I will find relief from the intensity and this means I'm releasing emotions stuck in my mind and body.

My gift is freedom from emotional intensity on whatever issue I'm working with. Now I have the space for new ways to see things to come into my experience.

I honor myself and my feelings more fully every time I consciously attend to them. This creates more emotional intelligence within me. Since tapping has a cumulative effect, I see there are many times where I catch myself before too much momentum gets created. I notice I can decide which feelings I will surf, and this is emotional freedom at its finest.

THOUGHT FOR THE DAY: Today I become more aware of my emotions and what they're trying to tell me.

January 3

"Feelings are just visitors, let them come and go." ~ Unknown

For me there are days, maybe even weeks and months, that quotes like this are cringe-worth for me. I get the point, but what we have here is a failure to communicate fully. Get my drift.

Here's my query: How? How do I let them come and go?

I want to let feelings come and go, but they can surprise me, more often than not. Just like yesterday's daily thoughts, it's the same here with a slight variation.

I can ponder that it's highly likely that I'm judging myself for not letting them come and go. I mean, I hear these pithy quotes often, and what happens is if I am judging myself and not aware of it, I feel bad about myself for not letting them come and go.

I'm not practiced at doing so. I wasn't encouraged to let feelings come and go; often whatever I was feeling was not okay. Sometimes I'm like a fly catcher for my emotions. They appear and I'm stuck to them like glue. I ruminate on them and they build momentum. What if this is okay? I ruminate on my emotions. I was virtually wired to do so.

What if, I can take this moment and just notice how I feel when I realize that it can be very challenging for me to let emotions come and go? What if I can notice the thoughts that tell me I "should" be able to do better? And what if I can pause and recognize that all the muck in my head is a series of thought patterns unknowingly practiced repeatedly. And what if, I can consider accepting the part of me that ruminates on thoughts in this moment and send myself a little more loving kindness? It's okay I do this. It is. And what if acceptance brings me relief and maybe even a little peace…right now.

THOUGHT FOR THE DAY: *What if I really am okay exactly as I am right now? No matter what.*

January 4

Every struggle in your life has shaped you into the person you are today. Be thankful for the hard times, they can only make you stronger...~ Daily Thought Quotes

When I read pithy quotes like this, how do I really feel? Do I feel good and nod in agreement? Or do I feel bad about myself because I'm NOT thankful for the hard times, especially when I'm in the thick of them.

It's highly likely that I am a product of the culture I've been raised in, where I'm told to be thankful for what's causing me pain, or to be grateful I don't have it worse. But where is my truth in this. My real truth. Not the truth I've been taught to manufacture with a smile that reveals sad eyes and my lot in life.

What if, like so many people I know, I got wired backwards?

What if, the biggest travesty to my well-being is NOT allowing myself the full expression of my truth, no matter how someone else might feel about it, including myself?

What if, tapping provides me the space to allow myself my unadulterated truth, no matter how inappropriate it may appear?

When I give myself the space, in a safe and healthy way, to tap through whatever is surfacing for me, I now can free myself from the shackles of being "appropriate" about my truth. Being appropriate can cause spiritual by-pass which merely glosses over emotions.

5

When I use tapping, I can allow myself to be as inappropriate as I need to be, in a safe and healthy way, so I have access to emotional liberation that's on the other side of acknowledging my truth about whatever is bothering me in any moment.

THOUGHT FOR THE DAY: _I can learn to allow myself my truth and my truth can set me free._

January 5

Always speak the truth, even if your voice shakes. ~ Bumper sticker

What if this was acceptable in my culture?

It is and it isn't. It is as long as it works for those hearing the truth. And it isn't for those who can't hear the truth.

But what if, I can give myself my truth, no matter what? When I tap on my truth, I can do this alone and allow myself the truth, the whole truth and nothing but the truth.

This is liberation in action. As I learn to do this, I am no longer bound by convention, or societal standards of what's appropriate or inappropriate. It's me with myself and my truth.

On the other side of my truth is emotional freedom and detachment from needing others to hear and know my truth, because I'm hearing it and honoring it in myself.

I'll have more of that please.

THOUGHT FOR THE DAY: *My unadulterated truth can set me free.*

January 6

Don't believe everything you think.
~Unknown

The bully in my brain (inner critic, ego) constantly parachutes into my life at the most inopportune times, filling me with fear, self-doubt, self-judgment, you name it. It fills my mind with all the things that could go wrong or won't work out and sends me into a tailspin of emotion which it has me circling the drain with my thoughts.

What if this is just a part of me as a human? An aspect of me. What if this bully in my brain is the culmination of the critical authority figures I've heard throughout my life?

What if I can catch this inner bully dumping manure into my psyche?

What if I can recognize that I can't stop my thoughts, but I can interrupt them?

If I think I have to stop negative thinking, I only pressurize myself to master a task that's actually impossible.

Let me try to stop the next thought that pops into my head. I might find a blank moment or two, but sure enough a thought comes to mind without me asking it too. It just comes.

What if today, I can set the intention to notice some of my thoughts and interrupt the ones I don't like? Interrupting is doable and it has a cumulative effect. It also takes pressure off of me, especially if I'm unknowingly bullying myself with the belief I should eradicate negative thoughts.

What a relief to know that I can interrupt what I can't stop?

THOUGHT FOR THE DAY: *I set the intention to interrupt my negative thoughts, when I notice them, knowing this is a big step in a more positive direction for me.*

January 7

Name your inner critic then tell him/her to shut up. ~ Pinterest

My inner bully can take on a demonic type vocabulary. It can be hideously macabre. It can be my own inner horror show. I may have heard it's trying to protect me, but I'm not so sure. This voice has people take themselves out of life on earth, so I'm not sure how this could be helpful.

When my inner bully is playing the horror show, I bet I can catch it occasionally and tell it to shut the hell up. I mean this is hell on earth, listening to this inner a-hole.

What if it becomes empowering to tell it to go away? It might creep back in, but the beauty is, there is no limit to how often I can tell it to go away. Then I run it instead of it running me. Can I get a Glory Hallelujah on this one?

Here's the sneaking part: Sometimes the bully in my brain sounds so reasonable and rational. It's not demonic. It sounds like it's trying to get me to act. It sounds like, '

"Well you really should call your mother."

"Be the first to forgive."

"Put your big girl or big boy pants on and just do it."

But here's the million-dollar question...

How do I feel when the rational reasonable bully version speaks and I'm not congruent with what it's directing me to do right now?

If I feel bad...well that's my clue that the bully is taking on this sneakier form...that's "just trying to help me."

Stick a fork in me, I'm done with this sort of help.

What if today I can distinguish which version my bully is using to communicate?

What if this awakens me to all the ways the bully in my brain bullies me?

THOUGHT FOR THE DAY: Today I can tell by how I feel who's running me show.

January 8

Lack of forgiveness causes almost all of our self-sabotaging behavior. ~ Mark Victor Hansen

---

What if it's really the lack of self-forgiveness that causes my self-sabotaging behavior?

What if I can learn how to forgive, accept, and eventually even love myself? That may feel like a big ask of myself, but what if this could be possible?

What could change for me? One way to discover it is to practice this. I can see what lack of self-forgiveness has done for me. Not so good.

I like that by learning to forgive myself first, something amazing could happen in my life.

How do I do this?

Once again, I catch myself getting down on myself using lack of forgiveness to do it. When I catch this, I can interrupt it and over time, I bet I'll notice that I'm less self-critical and more self-accepting. This naturally leads to self-love without me have to "try" to love myself more.

THOUGHT FOR THE DAY: Today I can interrupt the bully in my brain when it yammers in my ear. This has the power to change how I see myself each time I do this.

January 9

The pain of today is the victory of tomorrow.
~ strugglersala.com

What if I need not marry the concept that struggling is a necessity?

What if struggling is something the ego, inner critic or bully in my brain came up with?

> *"You have been criticizing yourself for years and it hasn't worked. Try approving of yourself and see what happens."* ~ Louise Hay

When I have a lot of momentum of thought criticizing myself...like years of it, it can feel like a daunting task to approve of myself. I may have tried this with affirmations or positive self-talk, yet the bully in my brain is so entrenched that my mind just doesn't believe the positive.

Here's where I make this easier for myself. I need not try to think positive or even try to say nicer, kinder things to myself. I can, however, use interrupting my thoughts once again and what if what happens, over time, is I naturally feel more positive towards myself. I naturally think better thoughts about myself.

How could this be?

What if, I was born intact with pure positive energy, self-esteem, and good will towards myself? What if this all just got covered over, like clouds moving over the sun, so now my pure positive energy isn't as available to my human self? What if this interrupting business is the simplest, easiest way to shift from self-criticism to self-approval?

I simple interrupt the critical self-talk, when I notice it, and over time, I notice the criticism softens and creates a space for the pure positive being I truly am to come shining through. I need not believe this yet, but I like that this could be possible.

THOUGHT FOR THE DAY: *Today I play the role of pattern interrupter. When I notice the bully in my brain is active, I interrupt it, ask it to leave, or just take a freaking break.*

January 10

If I was meant to be controlled, I would have come with a remote. ~OurMindfulLife.com

I live in a culture that teaches me what emotions are appropriate and what emotions are forbidden.

When I feel many emotions in the "forbidden zone?" I suppress a lot of these emotions. They become off limits.

This doesn't allow me the full expression of my humanity.

Why did I come into this life installed with this full palette of emotions?

Aren't they meant to be felt? What if they can be felt through to their completion with tapping? I find a safe and healthy way to allow myself the fullest expression of all of my emotions and in doing so, I heal. I know who I truly am, independent of the trappings of societies programming.

THOUGHT FOR THE DAY: *Today, I find a safe and healthy place to honor myself and the amazing emotions I came installed with. In doing so, I honor me and my humanness.*

January 11

I never thought I was a bully…until I listened to how I speak to myself. I think I owe myself an apology. ~ Whisper

---

If I ever take time to tune into my thinking, I see I can be so mean to myself. Of course I am. I grew up believing a lot of lies, about myself that feel like truths, but they're still lies.

Lies like:

I'm not good enough.

I don't have what it takes. I'll never make it.

If I pause and reflect on the thoughts that fire off in my mind, I might ask myself the following…

Good enough for what exactly?

Have what it takes to do what?

Make what?

What happened is I fell asleep to the truth of my being. Truths like, I was born brilliant. Born worthy and deserving of every good thing. I am making it. I'm here. I'm alive and despite the lies I learned to believe about myself, I sitting here reading this book with the likely intention of seeing myself in a different and better way than I see myself when I tune into the mean girl or boy within me.

THOUGHT FOR THE DAY: *Just for today, I will entertain the idea that I really am enough exactly as I am right now.*

January 12

Don't judge each day by the harvest you reap
but by the seeds that you plant.

~ Robert Lewis Stevenson

This is a lovely thought in theory, but in practice, it's a different journey.

I would love it if I judged each day by the seeds I've planted, but I live in a fast-paced, go get 'um tiger, if is going to be, it's up to me world. The society I live in reveres the "movers and the shakers" in this world.

I'm trying to shake off the cobwebs of programming that would have me doing the exact opposite of this quote. The programming that tells me I am what I do. I am what I have. I am how I look.

My current "reality" is that I'm somehow missing the boat on the reaping a harvest I see so many around me reaping. I live in a world where comparison is Queen. Where I judge my insides by others outside and always find myself wanting.

This is a set-up for failure in a world that loves action and doership. Sometimes I just want to lie on the grass and watch the clouds go by, but that's not being productive. It's sounding like Robert Lewis Stevenson, knew something profound that got lost in translation in this face-paced world.

What if I could tap through the beliefs to be productive and I have to reap a harvest that others would love to have? What if I could tap on the ideal, (and it is just an idea) that I have to make it happen?

What if by doing so, a space is created within me to see things differently than the way I was programmed to see things? Who knows what's possible when I see life through a different lens? I think I'd like to find out.

THOUGHT FOR THE DAY: *I set the intention to open to possibility. And the beauty is this intention is enough. The how can come to me.*

January 13

The important thing is to not stop questioning.
Curiosity has its own reason for existing. ~ Albert
Einstein.

"Curiosity killed the cat." This saying alone can program me to quake in my shoes at being curious.

I might minimize a saying like this, knowing that I've remained curious, or I might have fear around being curious, just because I've heard this saying enough to make an impact. Then maybe I've heard it said this way this. Curiosity killed the cat, but satisfaction brought is back."

Simple enough but it's highly possible that simple yet repetitive sayings like this affect me. Anything I hear enough can program beliefs within me. Whether this example applies or not, I've got a few, if not many, programs that run my show without my conscious knowledge. Tapping is a highly effective tool to help me free myself from both conscious and unconscious programming that can limit me.

As I release these programs my curiosity naturally comes to the forefront in my mind in a far freer and easier way. Once again, I create the space for possibilities to come with grace and ease.

THOUGHT FOR THE DAY: What if today, I can realize there are a lot of things I've heard in my life, that aren't true.

January 14

And those who were seen dancing were thought to be insane by those who couldn't hear the music. ~ Friedrich Nietzsche

Word Up!! I've felt this way most of my life. When I was a little kid, I bet I can remember some moment when those around me thought I was crazy. When I was a child, I knew the truth of my being. I just knew it. I may not remember that I knew it, but I did. I spent a lot of time, hearing a lot of things about how life should be. How I should be. Who I should be and on and on until I couldn't help but fall asleep to my higher self. The self that's not trapped by labels or directives.

Tapping can help me attend to the very human part of myself. The part that fell asleep to the most authentic part of me. As I attend to the human, programmed part of me, I find relief from the smoke and mirrors of the cultural programming I grew up in.

Suddenly, as the smoke clears, I feel the dancer within rise up from behind the cultural programming. I dance with my authentic self and it's possible that some around me might see me as crazy, but it won't matter then, because I've reconnected with my inner self where everything is fresh and possible.

THOUGHT FOR THE DAY: Today I begin the journey of reconnecting with my authentic self. The part of me that knows exactly who I am.

January 15

You were wild once. Don't let them tame you. ~ Isadora Duncan

---

What if this is a statement of truth, that's gotten lost in translation?

What if I'm meant to be wild and free? What if being wild and free got a bad rap in the society I live in. Wild and free means crazy and irresponsible in many circles. Being "appropriate" is revered.

Who says it's inappropriate to speak my truth, even if others see it differently?

Being appropriate is overrated. Now this doesn't mean the I go crazy on people and follow an in the brain on the mouth philosophy. Or maybe it does? The point is, I seek to find my truth. My way. My unique journey.

When I allow myself to release all the fodder around being appropriate, a new me emerges. I think for myself again. I compare less and just live and let live more. I clear up my own side of the fence being true to myself and this allows me to be wildly and authentically me. The world could miss out on yet another amazing human if I stay bogged down in what's appropriate.

I get to find my own way. Walk my own unique path. I get to share with the world the amazing unique being I have always been within. This is the greatest gift I can give to myself and to those around me. Me being me, opens the space for them to be them.

THOUGHT FOR THE DAY: *Today I am open to getting even a glimpse of the wild and free authentic self within me. I might just be surprised at how amazing and endearing this part of me.*

January 16

> *"We must train from the inside out. Using our strengths to attack and nullify weaknesses. It's not about denying a weakness may exist, but about denying it's right to persist. "*
>
> *~ Vince McConnell*

I've heard so many motivational quotes like this one. If I'm honest with myself, this exhausts me. It also feels like a fight. I've been pushing my whole life.

Pushing to overcome limitations. Pushing to succeed. Pushing. Pushing. Pushing.

If I'm honest with myself. The pushing might appear to work on some level. It might appear to get me what I think I want, but at what cost?

The personal develop world is riddle with pushing energy and overcoming weaknesses. This may sound reasonable. It may sound reasonable to say I want to be the best version of myself. I want to succeed in my life.

What if I already am the best version of myself? What if I success can mean something unique? What if I can see things in a new way, as I unhook from a societal standard of success that's been programmed into me?

What if it's not about trying harder, or reaching higher?

What if it's about learning to accept and eventually even love everything about myself, especially the parts of me I may deem weak, unlovable, or unacceptable? What if my weaknesses aren't weaknesses at all? They're actually character adaptations I learned early in life to cope and survive.

What if there isn't anything weak about me, therefore there's no reason to attack or nullify any parts of me? I may not believe this yet, but it sure sounds better than attacking and nullifying any part of me. My inner parts are similar to my organs, they're there for a reason, so I must need them. This is a kinder way to see myself.

THOUGHT FOR THE DAY: *Today, I set the intention to do at least one nice thing for myself. In this way, I'm practicing kindness towards myself.*

January 17

"Do or don't do. There is no try." ~Yoda

"Trying doesn't get it done." ~ *John Wayne*

What if Yoda and John Wayne are wrong? What if trying does do it? I may have tried and failed many things if I see it from the vantage point of the world I live in.

What if every time I try, I'm actually one step closer to the thing I'm trying for?

My inner child could sure use some loving kindness because this part of me can get very triggered when she/he hears trying is basically a waste of time.

What if trying does do it? I'll keep trying because I don't want to give up on myself. I may appear to fail often, but this is a wonderful thing. The ability to keep trying can get me to a place where I realize I'm just pushing the ego's agenda.

When I wake up to this, I can see that I'm not alone. If I tune into the Great Spirit, or whatever I prefer to call it, I can turn any challenge over to this power great than myself. When I do this, I actually open up to greater possibilities. Things now have a way to unfolding with a lot more ease. So trying can do it, eventually.

THOUGHT FOR THE DAY: *

January 18

"How would you nurture her if you were the mother of little you?" ~ *Kris Carr*

My wounded inner child wants to feel accepted and loved. It's a great question for me to ponder. How would I nurture my wounded inner child self?

As I ponder this, I might be guided in ways to really reparent my inner child and give to myself what I never got.

I give my wounded inner child a voice.

I listen to this part of me.

I honor this part of me.

I care of this part of me.

I'm present to this part of me.

I tap into and through anything my wounded inner child needs to.

What can change for me as I learn to nurture my wounded inner child?

I will answer this for myself. Only everything can change and for the better.

THOUGHT FOR THE DAY*: Today I can find one thing to do for my little self, so I practice accepting this nurturing and loving this part of me.*

January 19

I have so much to do that I will spend the first three hours in prayer.

~ Martin Luther King

Wow! This is amazing actually. It may not be prayer for me exactly. Maybe it's communing with something greater than myself that allows things to unfold in amazing and even magical ways.

So MLK spent three hours praying when he realized he had so much to do. What could happen for me, if I even spent 5 - 10 minutes first thing in the morning. To center myself and ground myself into a new reality. The reality there is a force in this human experience on my side.

If I've had a rough past around God, a Higher Power, or religion, I may not trust this idea.

The beauty is, I can acknowledge whatever I need to while tapping. As I do this, I can find relief and soothing from the anxiety, fear, overwhelmed and so much more.

I can follow Martin Luther King's lead and start my day with a victory and tune into whatever I believe to be God. I need not spend three hours a day doing so. I can tune in and ask for guidance and direction. Once I'm soothed, I have so much more space and access to guidance.

THOUGHT FOR THE DAY: *I'm not alone. A force loves me and guides and directs me. I just need to tune in to it.*

January 20

Happiness is the new rich. Inner peace is the new success. Health is the new wealth. Kindness is the new cool. ~ Syed Balki

---

I like it. More of this please. I can actually do a detox off of the worldly descriptions of what success means.

As I wake-up from the epic programming society floods my conscious and unconscious with, I can see things anew. I can decide for myself what success means. I put my physical and mental health first. I desire inner peace overall.

When I put the most important person in my life...me...first...I become kinder to myself. From this place, I find I am naturally kind to others, because I'm filling up my own cup first.

Society might tell me this is selfish. Society might tell me this is wrong. In more fragile moments, when the bully in my brain is feeding my lies, I might fall back to sleep and believe these lies about what makes me successful, rich, healthy, and free. When I catch myself in the act of believe a lie, I've made a huge step forward, because I am now observing this play out. This is where I have the power to tap and interrupt this programming and find relief from the lies.

In this relief, I now have access to the slower, creative, thinking part of my brain that opens up to new possibilities. I need not believe this yet, but I can experiment and see what comes. I might be abundantly and pleasantly surprised.

THOUGHT FOR THE DAY: *What if all I have to do today is interrupt my limiting thoughts, when I catch them? What if this is enough and what if this is a great beginning?*

January 21

"…the fucked-up part of it all is that even though she can hear her own heart breaking she's still willing to love the same one who broke it" ~ r.h. Sin

---

How often have I heard things like this? And how often does this leave me feeling worse about myself. I might be someone who's repeatedly "loved" someone who's 'done me wrong' or 'broken my heart' but something is missing in this. That something is compassion.

Having compassion for the wounded child in me that would sell her/his very soul to find something remotely resembling love is a big step towards liberating myself from the character adaptations I've acquired over the years to survive.

When I continue to treat myself with self-recrimination, I'm doomed to repeat the patterns I'd swear, on all that is holy, that I want to release.

This is often why I stay stuck in a cycle of failing. It's the judgement of self that holds so many patterns in place in my life. The personal development world will likely tell me I need to be different. I need to Get Off My Ass (The Law of GOYA) and effect lasting change. This also discourages and disappoint me.

I can ask myself the following question and then seek inside for the answer.

(Not seek the outside world for the answer.)

Here goes: Has being hard on myself, pushing myself, demanding more from myself and judging myself EVER allowed me to create graceful, peaceful, uplifting, lasting change?

THOUGHT FOR THE DAY: *What if I can catch the pushing, demanding verbiage I hear as a reflection of my inner bully attempting to run my show, even once today?*

January 22

---

*"You'll become happy when you stop reacting
and start controlling your emotions." ~
KushanDWizdom*

Ok now...Hahahahahaha!!! Really? Good freaking luck!

Controlling my emotions has been one of the biggest problems in my life. As if I'm meant to control them in a world that teaches me to deny and suppress emotions. This is when emotions become forbidden. These emotions are off limits, and these are okay to feel. Please!!!

I was born this this amazing palette of emotions all meant to be felt. Why would they be in me anyway. Emotions only become out of control when they've had to be suppressed repeatedly, in a world uncomfortable with them.

What if this is all just wrong? What if tapping allows my this safe, private, highly effective way to allow my emotions to be what they are? When I tap on my truth...whatever that truth may be, I free these stuck emotions from my nervous system. The beauty of doing this is, over time, I find I'm naturally more content and able to exhibit emotional intelligence without "trying" to control anything.

THOUGHT FOR THE DAY: *Feeling fully frees me when I do so in a safe and healthy way. Tapping provides me this way.*

January 23

> *"Holding onto anger is like drinking poison and expecting the other person to die."*
>
> ~ *Buddha*

Am I actually about to argue with The Buddha? No, I'm not. I actually agree with Buddha, but sometimes my wounded child gets so activated that I do hang on to anger. But what's behind me holding on to anger?

I might believe that I'm letting the other person off the hook for their offenses if I don't remain angry. With tapping, I don't have to 'try' to let go of my anger. With tapping, I get to go into the anger and feel it fully and allow it to do what it's meant to do…move through me.

If I suppress the feeling of my anger with the belief, I shouldn't feel what I'm feeling, then guess what? Anger can consume me.

When I allow space for my anger, in a safe and healthy way, the anger moves on. It doesn't stay stuck in my body. If I can remember that "feelings aren't buried dead, they're buried alive." (Janice Berger) I'm encouraged to feel my anger or any other emotion, so I can be free of the ties that bind me to my emotions.

THOUGHT FOR THE DAY: *As I allow space for my anger with tapping, I have a tool that can set me free.*

January 24

"A clear understanding of negative emotions dismisses them." ~ Vernon Howard

---

Can I get a hell yeah on this? And can I add tapping to this recipe so I can actually understand what's beneath my negative emotions?

What's beneath my negative emotions is actually my truth.

My truth does have the power to set me free. My truth, when addressed with the tool of tapping, allows me to see my negative emotions so differently.

I understand what fuels them and where they came from and why they show up when they do. The more understanding I have about any emotion the more I find compassion for myself.

Self-compassion is the building block of true and lasting change within me.

THOUGHT FOR THE DAY: *There are no bad or wrong emotions. There are just emotions. Some feel better to feel than others, but all of my emotions are telling me something that can help me.*

January 25

"Inner peace begins the moment you choose not to allow another person or event to control your emotions." ~ EyeOpenerQuotes.com

This is so true.

I know I am free when an event that might normally set me reeling no longer does. I know I am free when a someone can say something that might be harsh, insensitive, or potentially hurtful and I merely shrug and think, "They must be having a bad day."

But HOW…how do I get to this unicorns ridden by fairies island? The place in the stratosphere where I'm not affected by someone else's pettiness or a challenging event.

Yep…I tap tap tap. I use tapping and "go deep" to catch what's being passed to me.

I allow myself all of my hurt, anger, rage, feelings of injustice, fear, and the beat goes on. Any emotions that surface are ripe for the picking. I get to use tapping to give every emotion it's day in court. To expound, to lament my woes is me-ness. I get to be a drama queen or kind extraordinaire.

Once I've tapped through every nook and cranny of my emotions, as best I can, or supported by a seasoned professional, I can feel freer.

I can also remember this is a process.

It's not as if I'm going to never get triggered again.

The last time I checked, I'm still in this body and still having this human experience. Along with my humanness are people and events I can sometimes want to kick to the curb. And I may. But I am reminded that my truest freedom of all, are the stolen moments when I notice I am free of other opinions. I notice I'm free to witness events that can send me to the corner with my blankie and pacifier, without being negatively affected this time. I anchor in these moments as wins because they are.

THOUGHT FOR THE DAY: *I set the intention to anchor in the little wins I have during this day. And they are there for me to see.*

January 26

The loudest voice isn't the truest voice. ~
Unknown

This is good to ponder. As I pay attention to my thoughts, it's highly likely I will go through a phase where I hear the mental chatter that just rambles on between my ears. If I'm feeling bad, I can be sure this is the bully in my brain, doing due diligence and filling my head with everything that won't work and why it won't work and how I'm not capable. Urgh!!!

I might also notice that when I'm highly emotionally charged, this is my wounded inner child trying to get some attention.

Here's the breakdown:

The Bully in my brain is this punitive, authoritative voice that loves to tell me what to do and what's wrong with me and the situation. It can sound demonic in tone or it can be sneaky and sound reasonable. I know it's the bully by how I feel. If I feel bad about myself, it's a guarantee the bully is running a rampage champaign in my head.

The Wounded Child is emotionally charge. It can be swimming in a pool of emotion that often create, fear, panic, and anxiety in me.

The Bully beats up on the child and the child gets saturated in emotion.

Here's the magic in the awareness of who's running my show. These are both loud voices that take over but neither of these voice cares with it the truth of me. These two parts of me learned to believe lies from the outer world and these lies are actually crazy. They may feel true and be loud, but they are not the truth of me.

The truth of me is so much greater than allow the thoughts that flow through my head. When I know who's running my show, I separate from these parts of me. This allows the space for me to hear my authentic, healthy self.

The authentic, healthy self knows everything will be okay. It knows I'm worthy and deserving of every good thing, just because I am. It's my true nature. It's the part of me a fell asleep to in this crazy world. As I continue recognize the bully and the wounded child, they lose the ability to run my show. Now my authentic self can shine through.

THOUGHT FOR THE DAY: *Today I tune in to see who's running my show.*

January 27

---

*"Time is precious. Make sure you spend it
with the right people." ~ Emotional Quotes*

This is great in theory, to make sure I spend my precious time with the right people. But HOW do I do this? Especially when I may not have been raised to choose the "right" people.

What if there's a more expanded awareness around this?

I might find that I'm around people who annoy the hell out of me and if I walk away from every single person that annoys, hurts, frustrates, or bothers me, I might find myself on fantasy island with those fairies riding unicorns.

I'm in a body for a reason. I'm in human form for a reason. I'm here to learn a few things. If I systematically eliminate every other human displeasing to me, I'm actually limiting what's possible for me.

What if the people in my life in any moment are there by design to help my soul evolve? What if I came into this lifetime with a soul contract and part of that was being around people who trip me up and trigger me, so I can learn how to not be so triggered around them? What if they are my greatest teachers because they are so challenging for me?

This does not mean I roll over and "take it." It means I see these people in a new way. I see them as revealers to what shows me the places within that I am seeking to evolve. What if I can learn to trust that when our time together is complete, I will know and I will move on without angst and anger and hurt. It will just be time to move on.

This is a different way to see the "right" and the "wrong" people.

THOUGHT FOR THE DAY: *What if every single person in my life is actually there to reveal or to teach my soul something it's chosen to learn?*

January 28

"The goal isn't to get rid of all of your negative thoughts and feelings; that's impossible. The goal is to change your response to them." ~ *Marc and Angel Hack Life*

Word Up!!! Yes. Yes and Yes. What a relief to know that it's actually impossible to get rid of all of my negative thoughts and feelings. It's so true. When I get this, I can stop trying to think positive. To stop trying to be positive. To stop trying to just think happy thought so everything will be okay. I will say this again. What at freaking relief!

I need not stop my thoughts. I can't but with tapping I can interrupt them. This is doable. I can interrupt thoughts that don't serve me before they have my circling the drain down into a black hole of negativity.

The key is, when I notice my thoughts are negative, I can interrupt them with tapping. The beauty is I will not notice them all the time but even a little is enough to effect change.

Noticing and interrupting them is like putting a scratch on an old vinyl record. The song will never sound the same with the scratch in it. Thus my thoughts change the more I interrupt my negative thoughts. They lose their momentum and over time, I find that my thoughts naturally become more positive, because my authentic self has the space to be heard.

Over time, I will notice that my resting thought rate is infinitely more positive. This is evidence that I'm actually changing my physiology, by changing the neurochemicals that flood my cells.

THOUGHT FOR THE DAY: I can't stop my negative thoughts, but I can interrupt them when I catch them.

January 29

"Speak when you are angry, and you will make the best speech you'll ever regret."

~ Unknown

Anger can be both healthy and unhealthy. Anger in its healthy form gives me the ability to set boundaries, to speak my truth, to stand up for what I believe in and so much more.

Anger in its unhealthy form will have my making a speech I later regret. If I'm reading this, I can be reminded that I am human. And along with being human comes both healthy and unhealthy displays of anger.

When I own my humanity and own that I will always be a work in progress, I can find more of that amazing self-compassion so necessary for true lasting change. I may make more speeches when I'm triggered that I later regret. If I do, I have this amazing opportunity to practice more self-acceptance and forgiveness. I suspect I can always use more practice with both of these.

When I forgive myself for my humanness, my sincere and heartfelt apologize can open the heart of another in amazing ways. I can give out what I now find within myself. Compassionate acceptance of all that is so very human about me.

THOUGHT FOR THE DAY: *All is well.*

January 30

"The biggest issue with humans is they do not know how to handle their thoughts and emotions." ~ Sadhguru

True and yet of course this is true. If I'm reading this, it's highly likely that I was not shown how to handle my thoughts and emotions. I live and grew up in a world that would prefer I suppress my emotions. Most people have been taught that their strong because they don't appear to express emotions. They go through tough circumstances and are revered for

"Keeping that stiff upper life."

"Big boys don't cry."

"There's no crying in baseball."

These attitudes are everywhere.

Tapping allows me to access suppressed emotions. And what a gift this is. To learn how to feel fully. A true gift, no matter what the world tells me.

When I learn to access and feel more fully, I become someone who is more emotionally fit. What this does for me is allows me to be a human who does know how to handle my thoughts and emotions a little better every day.

THOUGHT FOR THE DAY: *I am learning to become emotionally fit.*

January 31

---

*"If you know how to handle your thoughts
and emotions there will be no such thing as*

anxiety, stress or tension for you." ~ Sadhuguru
quotes

Hmmm! Is this possible in this body, having this human experience. If I interrupt the thoughts that disrupt my life and my world, I find relief. It feels like a big promise there will be no such thing as anxiety, stress, or tension for me. I mean the world I live in is a fast-paced, make it happen kinda world.

I get programmed every day, depending on what I'm viewing to be more, reach higher, set goals, become who I'm meant to be. Stick a fork in my, I'm done with this nonsense. And it is nonsense.

I want to learn how to accept and then maybe even embrace all of my thoughts and emotions. Allow them to do what they are intended to do. Move through me to their completion...for this moment.

An hour from now, I could be in a stewpot of anxiety, stress and tension and if I'm suggesting to myself that I will arrive and cross over some intended finish line of that permanently completes me...is that movie line...you complete me? Nope, it's just me learning to embrace the fullness of what it means to be in a body on planet earth.

I may find tremendous relief from anxiety, stress, and tension, but I can be guaranteed that something in life on this planet will happen again that can trigger these. Tapping is a technique that can help me move through these emotions and be less afraid and more confident that I won't get swallowed up by my thoughts and emotions.

THOUGHT FOR THE DAY: *I am a wonderful work in progress.*

February

February 1

> *"Spend your time on those that love you unconditionally. Don't waste it on those who only love you when the conditions are right for them." —Buddha*

The problem with this idea is that, if I'm honest with myself, I don't think I actually know anyone who loves me unconditionally, and it's highly likely that I'm not unconditionally loving towards anyone, either (other than, perhaps, my dog or cat if I have one, but even these beings can drive me bananas occasionally).

As long as I'm in this body, on this planet, in this culture, I will likely be conditional with people—even my children. It's part of the human experience.

I suspect I wouldn't be on this planet in the first place if I were truly unconditionally loving towards others, and those that I love would be someplace else, too, if they were truly unconditionally loving. That's a big ask.

What if I could acknowledge that unconditional love comes from a world run by the ego? Unconditional love is wonderful in theory, but I suspect it might take me a few more lifetimes to acquire this saint-like status.

So for now, it might be immensely helpful if I cut myself some slack and understand that I can walk away from people when I know it's time to, but I can continue to learn and grow when I and those I love are being conditional.

THOUGHT FOR THE DAY: *What if it's enough I know that I want to be more loving and I will continue to practice this?*

February 2

"Stop letting people who do so little for you control your mind, feelings and emotions." —*Will Smith*

What's missing here? Oh, I know. How? How do I stop doing this?

I probably have to keep bumping up against feeling controlled by others over and over again before it registers that I'm allowing others to control me. It's likely this is a long-held pattern.

If I do find I go to an apple tree for orange juice again and again, what helps me most is to understand there is always a very good, unconscious reason I do this. This reason is always always always a misinformed way I'm attempting to protect myself.

It worked when I was a kid on some level. And I had to figure out how to adapt to my circumstances, without guidance and direction from the adults around me.

How do I know this? I know this if I am going to people who give me little when I give so much. I know this because I get triggered by someone else's crazy behavior and I take it on and take it personally. I do this because I learned to do that early in life.

My early imprinting was going to an empty well to fill up. I wasn't taught it was an inside job and I wasn't taught how to access this part of me. I was taught to lose touch with my authentic self. My healthy self.

It's through dealing with feeling controlled by someone else that allows me to see the pattern and keep interrupting it. Eventually, I learn a new way. A healthier way. A way that includes my wellbeing.

THOUGHT FOR THE DAY*: The sticky people in my life are often in my life to help wake me up to a better way of being.*

February 3

> "Try your best not to cry or go into rage after someone criticizes you in the smallest way." —HealthyPlace.com

I may have tried this and had little to no success, resulting in me feeling worse than I did before. The truth is I can try to not cry or go into a rage all day long, but if I'm not attending to the underlying reasons I am crying or going into a rage, all my trying will do is make me feel worse about myself.

Tapping shortcuts the "trying" game. Trying can help, but if I'm forcing myself to sit on my hands or keep my mouth shut, this only buries more emotions in my body. This negatively affects me mentally, emotionally, and physically, especially the more I try and fail.

Tapping gets to the heart of the matter; the hidden reasons below the surface as to why I cry, or why I become enraged, or both.

Tapping short circuits the patterns that have been in place for many years that. It allows the unconscious to become conscious. When I see what triggers me to cry or feeling enraged, and tap through this, I find relief. I notice that I'm capable of pausing first, and then responding, rather than just reacting with tears and rage. I'm becoming more emotionally fit.

THOUGHT FOR THE DAY: *Unless I'm shown the 'how to,' I'll just have to pass.*

February 4

> *"Please don't expect me to always be good, kind and loving. There are times when I will be cold and thoughtless and hard to understand." —@therandomvibez*

Hallelujah! This is an example of giving myself permission to not be perfect. It's permission to, occasionally, lose myself in emotions when I get triggered.

Perfectionism kills my humanity. It doesn't allow for the amazing complexities of my human existence to exist. When I hold myself to impossible standards, everything becomes impossible.

I came installed with a fully loaded, amazing palette of emotions meant to be felt fully. This concept, however, becomes problematic in a society that reveres suppression; a society that tells me I'm strong if I control myself and control my emotions.

The only reason emotions get out of control is because they aren't felt in the moment. They are suppressed and, when suppressed, they eventually have to go somewhere.

Maybe the next time I lose myself in my emotions, I can remind myself this is a by-product of suppressing them. They have to go somewhere, and at that moment, the lid just came off. I just couldn't contain them anymore. My bullshit meter exploded and so did my emotions.

What if the more I learn to allow myself to feel fully, in a safe and healthy way (tapping can provide me with this way), my emotions become more regulated? I would find more moments where I could allow myself my truth and my feelings, and I would become more emotionally fit because I could honor my emotions in the moment.

THOUGHT FOR THE DAY: *If I lose myself in my emotions, I'm still a good person. It's just showing me that there's more to feel and release.*

February 5

"One great lesson I learned from my life…there is no market for your emotions, so never advertise your feelings, just show your attitude." —Nishan Panwar

---

This quote comes from a world that programs us that emotions are just not okay. There's a host of emotions that end up on the forbidden list, meaning you shouldn't feel them or display them.

What if this is just plain wrong?

As I learn to release the forbidden (i.e., off-limit) emotions and allow them into my experience, I actually learn the richness in these emotions. As I realize there isn't a single emotion that's bad or wrong, there are just emotions, this can level the playing field for me.

It's not the emotion that is bad, it's the actions that come from the suppression of emotions that can cause harm. So doesn't it stand to reason then that feeling fully is advisable and actually necessary for my mental, emotional, and physical health and well-being?

As I release stuck emotions, I clear the space in myself to learn how to feel fully and be freed. I move on from emotions so much faster. I harbor fewer resentments. I genuinely and easily let go of anger without having to try to let it go. I'm able to let go without shaming myself about any emotion I feel because I'm no longer making them wrong, forbidden, or off-limits.

Liberation and freedom are the other side of feeling fully.

THOUGHT FOR THE DAY*: As I learn to feel fully, I liberate myself, my body, my mind, and my spirit.*

February 6

"*What's most important in animation is
the emotions and the ideas being portrayed.
I'm a great believer of energy and emotion.*"
—Ralph Bakshi

Talk to any actor and they will tell you that it's the ability to emote that makes a character believable; emotions communicate everything in acting. An actor can melt into the role they are playing when they can display and convey the character's emotions effectively.

I can learn a lot from this.

What if I can learn to allow myself my emotions the way actors allow for the expression of their characters' emotions? I get better at doing this effectively with practice and using tapping to go deeper into the emotions buried in my body for years. This is a great first step.

Learning how to effectively free my body and mind from buried emotions gives me the ability to become emotionally fit. This allows me to react less and respond more from an emotionally intelligent place.

The more I release, the freer I feel, and the more emotional intelligence I'm able to access.

THOUGHT FOR THE DAY: What if I can notice what emotions I'm feeling at different times during the day?

February 7

"If you focus on the hurt, you will continue to suffer. If you focus on the lesson, you will continue to grow."
—*HealthyPlace.com*

This idea can trip me up. I get this is true and is actually great advice, but what's missing for me once again is how? How do I do this when I'm riddled with hurt?

I feel the hurt.

I can use tapping to go deeper into the hurt and to give presence to the hurt.

Tapping helps me to allow the hurt to be felt more fully so it can ultimately be released. I will then find I feel lighter and freer because I've allowed space for my hurt and felt it fully. I find I'm less afraid or judgmental of my emotions because I've allowed them space to exist.

I see now that I've been taught the opposite of this in the world I live in. Suppression never works. It just sets the stage for an emotional blow up, and when I blow up emotionally, I often feel bad about myself.

If I can understand that the blow ups have to happen when the suppression of emotions is involved, I might be a little kinder to myself. I might learn to forgive myself because I understand why it's happening, and thus understand the huge benefit of fully feeling my hurt (or any other emotion) fully.

When I do this, the "lesson" doesn't have a bitter taste in my mouth. New awareness helps me see things in a better way.

THOUGHT FOR THE DAY: *What if today I can practice feeling one emotion a little more fully while tapping?*

February 8

"If you never heal from what hurt you, then you'll bleed on people who didn't cut you." —NotSalmon.com

True, true, and true. I don't mean to bleed on people who didn't cut me, but here's another perspective: often the people in my life are mirrors that reflect back the healed and the unhealed parts within me.

If I see things this way then each person in my life, no matter how maddening, can become a teacher. Not in a punishing, I've got another life lesson to deal with, but in a soul evolving way.

What if my soul and those around me came into this human experience knowing what was needed for our evolution? What if our souls knew each other when we met, and knew we would dance with each other so we can evolve?

48

What if the most challenging people in my life, those people who might seem to never understand me, are the greatest revealers for me? They play their part, and I play my part to evolve.

It's a different perspective for sure. And maybe it's true.

THOUGHT FOR THE DAY: *What if I can entertain the idea that the people in my life are all there by design for my evolution?*

February 9

"Heavy hearts, like heavy clouds in the sky are best relieved by the letting of a little water." —Christopher Morley

That's what I'm talking about. The letting of a little, or maybe even a lot of emotions. Emotions suffocated for years. This has the power to bring incredible relief.

I learn that I no longer have to bite my lip or hold my tongue. I find a safe and healthy place to allow the fullest expression of my truth—the unadulterated truth—and I put "being appropriate" on the shelf for the moment. At the end of it all, the person or situation I'm upset about might never have to hear any of my unadulterated truth; I at least get to give this to myself.

Once I've allowed myself this gift, what I often find on the other side is the freedom to express myself to someone in a far more emotionally intelligent way. This is such a blessing.

I get to get all the angst, hurt, sadness, and heaviness of buried emotion out of my body. I get to free myself from the burden of this heaviness and, as I do this, I set myself free.

THOUGHT FOR THE DAY: *What if today I can find some time to allow myself my unadulterated truth in a safe and healthy space? Emotional liberation and freedom can then be mine.*

February 10

"Great salespeople [don't] have the ability to feel sorry for themselves."
—Barbara Corcoran

Come on now! You mean to tell me there's never, in the history of time, been a great salesperson that hasn't felt sorry for themselves at some point? Please. This is definitely a product of a culture that's highly attached to the constraints of the ego.

If you're in a body, you're subject to many emotions and experiences, and feeling sorry for yourself is one of them.

There's so much momentum around not allowing yourself to feel sorry for yourself. But my wounded inner child is riddled in feeling sorry for themself. When I was child I couldn't run away, so I had to figure out how to adapt. This part of me needs a fuller, freer expression.

In fact, I will bake a cake and buy party hats and balloons. I might even buy my inner child a present and say, "Have at it. This is your epic pity party.

You finally get the chance to begin expressing just how sorry for yourself you feel."

And guess what? When you do this, you will come to a place where you release the feeling of being sorry for yourself. You might have to revisit this pity party at other times in your life, but that's okay because now you know how to get to the other side of self-pity as opposed to staying stuck in it.

In this way, I get to give my victimized inner child their truth and the truth will set this part of me free.

THOUGHT FOR THE DAY: What if I can give fuller expression to the wounded, victimized child in me without the judgement?

February 11

"The wound is the place where the light enters you." —Rumi

What a lovely way to see my wounds. My wounds have the power to shape who I become.

Maybe I know different people that have gone through very similar circumstances and one of those people grew from it while the other person seemed to lose themselves to it. Why would this be?

What if it's closely related to the allowing of emotions? Allowing the full expression of every emotion that surfaces and giving it the space to be honored?

What if one of them used the wound as the place where they ultimately let the light enter them? What if the other person was so entrenched in the beliefs of the world they grew up because they just didn't know how to allow the light in? They might have continued down a path that lacked self-compassion and judged themselves harshly, ultimately remaining stuck in the should haves or the shouldn't haves.

Self-compassion is so important to my well-being, and yet it's amazing how the world I live in can seem to prefer giving honor to being hard on myself. This is such a misguided approach to effecting lasting change.

The beauty is that I'm waking up from the nightmare of this crazy programming, and self-compassion is becoming a very important practice for me (and it does take practice).

THOUGHT FOR THE DAY: *What if today I can be mindful of gifting myself some self-compassion?*

February 12

"The privilege of a lifetime is being who you are." —Joseph Campbell

What if I could actually learn to believe this is true and take it to heart? Perhaps I'll even practice treating myself with even just a little more love and respect.

Had I been told the truth of my being right from the start, I would already know that I deserve to be good to myself, to love myself, to nurture myself, to cherish myself, and to honor myself just because of the simple fact that I exist. This is my divine birthright.

I would already know not to punish or be hard on (or even sometimes just flat out mean) to myself. These are all concepts of a world deeply embedded in the consciousness of the ego.

Many institutions (which are man-made, thus inherently ego-based) teach me that being hard on myself will somehow effect true change within me.

I live in a world actually wired backwards; many things are the opposite of what I've been programmed to believe. When I realize this, I start to wake-up more fully each and every day.

When I learn to treat myself with more loving kindness, I learn how to be true to myself. I actually learn what's best for me. In this way, I learn the privilege of being my authentic self.

THOUGHT FOR THE DAY*: I am meant to love and accept myself. What if today is a great day to practice loving and accepting all parts of me?*

February 13

---

*"To accept ourselves as we are means to
value our imperfections as much as our
perfections." —Sandra Bierig*

I love the idea of accepting all parts of me. It's not something I learned how to do well, if at all, growing up.

The world of personal development often tells me to eradicate my limited thinking. It tells me to control my emotions and work hard to do it. If I'm unable to do these things, how do I feel? It's highly likely that I will feel bad about myself, and if I'm feeling bad about myself, I'm not accepting all of me or valuing what could be called my imperfections.

It takes practice to see aspects of myself that I don't care for and learned to accept them anyway (maybe even laugh at them). Learning to understand that I have a lot of momentum of thinking around rejecting my imperfections is helpful.

What if my so-called imperfections are character adaptations I learned to help me cope in life? That may sound crazy, but what if every imperfection has within it an unconscious pattern I learned that's attempting to protect myself? If I considered this as a possibility, could I find a little more acceptance for my imperfections?

As an example, could procrastination be a way I've learned to protect myself from being seen and a means to avoid potential criticism? Could eating those donuts be a way to soothe and comfort myself?

If I can practice seeing my imperfections as unconscious character adaptations I learned to protect myself, it may become more possible for me to ease into accepting all of me.

THOUGHT FOR THE DAY*: Today I will practice noticing when I do something that makes me cringe and ask myself, "If I had to guess, what is my reason for doing this?"(Notice what follows the "I do this because" and tap through that.)*

February 14

"Loving yourself is healing the world." —Jaymie Gerard

On this Valentine's Day, a day that can have so many people feeling lonely and like they're not enough, what if I can give myself the gift of loving myself?

How? How do I do this?

What if a great place to start is to write a down three things I like about myself? (Even if I have to squeeze them out.) I can notice the "yeah, buts" that might pop-up as I write these 3 things down, but that's great because the "yeah, buts" are my roadmap for what to tap on.

The "yeah, buts" may sound like this:

"Yeah, I'm a good cook, but remember that time you burnt that cake?"

"Yeah, I'm a good friend, but remember that time you weren't such a good friend?"

"Yeah, I'm loyal, but remember those times you gossiped?"

What comes after the "yeah, buts" is a view into my beliefs. The "yeah, buts" create an inner argument that keeps the status quo in place. This makes self-compassion, and thus loving myself, challenging when I believe what follows the "but" in my mind.

Now that I know what follows my "yeah, buts," I can tap so I find relief, which opens me up to self-compassion and self-love.

THOUGHT FOR THE DAY: What if today I can tune into my "yeah buts" and tap to soothe them, so compassion and love includes me?

February 15

"Losers quit when they fail. Winners
fail until they succeed." —Robert Kiyosaki

This is a classic example of how coaches or mentors in the personal development world can unknowingly (or knowingly) shame people, and it misses the point. There's no space to go below the surface as to why I don't appear to have the attributes of being a "winner."

When I believe in the concepts of winners and losers, I am believing the bully in my brain. I'm believing in separation rather than communion, competition rather than cooperation. This only makes me feel bad because

I'm either a winner or a loser. It actually objectifies me and ignores the multidimensional being I am.

I live in a culture that promotes thinking in terms of winners and losers—successful people and unsuccessful people. No wonder I can get caught up in this.

How do I know I'm caught up in the worldly culture that pushes the ego's agenda? I know by how I feel. When I feel bad, it's a great indicator that the bully in my brain is activated and my inner child is feeling powerless.

As I learn to realize who's running my show—the bully, the wounded child, or my healthy authentic self—I become able to choose who's allowed to keep talking.

Tapping is my ally because it helps me find relief from the potent emotions that get stimulated by the thoughts that create these emotions. As I soothe my emotions, I now have access to the healthy, authentic part of me.

The healthy authentic part of me has an entirely different perspective than the world that pushes the ego's agenda. The healthy authentic part of me never believes in winners or losers. It shows me the amazing being I am, below the muck the world feeds me.

THOUGHT FOR THE DAY: *Today I can have moments where I will notice who's running my show: the bully, the wounded child, or my healthy authentic self.*

February 16

"Failure is only the opportunity to begin again more intelligently." —Henry Ford

---

What a nice way to see failure. The perception of failure lets me know I'm active in life.

The long spoken of analogy about babies learning to walk is a great example here. Babies might get frustrated when they're first trying to walk; they might even throw a tantrum because of it, but when the tantrum passes, they get up and try again.

Then, one day, they're suddenly putting steps together that get them across the room. They might still stumble and have to get back up, but the day eventually comes where one foot goes consistently in front of the other, and now they are a walking human. A whole new world opens up for them.

The same can be said for me in my progress as a human on this planet. Each time I fail, I learn something I need to, and I become more emotionally intelligent.

I have fallen, gotten frustrated, and thrown my own temper tantrums, but this is part of the human condition. I bet if I look I can often find where I've initially failed at something, but then a day comes where I overcome the supposed failure and the stars align just right and I've now changed a pattern in my life for the better.

There might also be those things that don't seem to change much. I may have tapped on these things more times than I can count, but I still see no visible change for the better. What if this is just letting me know it could be time to turn this over to whatever I believe would or could be a supportive higher being?

What if, as I learn that surrendering to this "thing," it's actually a way of reminding myself that I'm not alone? Are there forces at work here that have my back and support me? I just need to remember this and continue to come back to this idea.

What if this thing that has caused me pain and suffering is the very thing that reconnects me to this source?

THOUGHT FOR THE DAY: *If something is not changing, what if it's time to practice surrendering to whatever I believe in and I begin again?*

February 17

> *"Learning starts with failure, the first failure is the beginning of education."*
> *—John Hersey*

What if I had been taught this idea that mistakes are okay? What if I had been encouraged to always make new mistakes? I would likely be kinder and gentler with myself had I actually been encouraged to believe that what appears to be failure is actually the way I learn.

I do learn from my mistakes. I might make the same mistakes over and over again for a while, but this too is part of the learning curve.

If I keep making the same mistakes multiple times, I can get down on myself about it. But I likely have patterns of thinking that have been in place for years, even decades, and when this is the case it makes complete sense there are things I bump up against repeatedly. Each time I do, if I'm aware of it and interrupt the pattern, I get closer to a different result.

I may not see much evidence right away because often the shifts in my thinking aren't visible for a while. The work that's happening is on the inside.

The more I tap, the more it has a cumulative effect. With consistency, I'll notice the subtle little shifts that are evidence that things are shifting for me.

I am working from the inside out. I'm actually changing the expression of my genes each time I do this. The day will come where I become aware of a significant change in my behavior, but the truth is the consistent little shifts have created what appears to be a big shift.

THOUGHT FOR THE DAY*: What if today I can set the intention to notice the little wins I experience?*

February 18

"If "Plan A" didn't work the alphabet has 25 more letters!" —quotereel.com

Glory Hallelujah! Another great reminder I can always begin again. I might have to take a break and regroup, but this is honoring me.

I get to do a do-over any time I'm ready to. Time will pass regardless, so why not try again, if I feel the intuitive impulse? (Not the pushing energy of the ego.)

Another option could be that it's time to move on to an entirely new plan.

When things don't appear to work out for me, could it be possible that I'm actually being guided and directed to something that's even better for me? Something that my simple human self can't see or imagine. Could it be possible that there's so much more available when I'm open to the possibility of it?

This is a nicer way to see my circumstances, when I've tried hard to make a change and it just doesn't seem to happen. Otherwise, I can keep beating myself up with thoughts like:

"I'm not doing this right."

"I'm not thinking positively enough."

"I need to visualize more."

I think I like this idea a lot, that if somethings not working out for me, it's not meant to. I think I'll ponder this idea more. I bet I'll find relief from the troubling thoughts that can overtake me. Once I've done this, I can begin again from an entirely new place and open to what comes.

THOUGHT FOR THE DAY: *What if today I can consider that not everything I want is for my highest good because there's something better for me lining up?*

February 19

"*My great concern is not whether you have failed, but whether you are content with your failure.*" —*Abraham Lincoln*

The idea that I could actually become content when things don't work out for me—to be content in the face of something not "going my way" —is a paradigm shift. What if this means there are greater possibilities for me?

When I find myself upset that there's something I've appeared to fail at, I can tap to find relief from the pain of my "failing." When I find relief from it, I create the space to see failing in a new way.

I open up to the possibility that the things I think I want may not be for my highest and best good. When I do this, I become open for new things to come rather than me thinking I have to figure it all out on my own.

What if things work so much better for me?

What a concept.

THOUGHT FOR THE DAY: *What if today I can entertain the idea that there are things so much better for me as I learn to let go of my agenda (the ego's agenda, actually)*

February 20

"I've failed over and over and that is why I succeed." —Michael Jordan

---

The master of basketball, a man seen as the most successful basketball player of all time, is telling me he succeeded because he failed so much.

I live in a world that pushes success in a very materialistic way. For example, think of the advertising I'm exposed to. The images often include: the car I drive, the house I live, the kids I have, the relationship(s) I have, or the physical wealth I have.

What if I can release the idea that these things make me successful? What if my failure is my guidance to what's next for me? I can tap and interrupt that bullying voice in my head that fills me with inadequacy and hopelessness. As I find relief, I might be able to see failing in a new way, and what if I eventually learn to define what success means to me independent of the world's view of success?

This can be a new beginning for me.

THOUGHT FOR THE DAY: *What if today I can discover my own voice around failing and success and what it means for me?*

February 21

"Develop success from failures.
Discouragement and failure are two of the
surest steppingstones to success." —Dale
Carnegie

Dale Carnegie was a pioneer in what is now known as the personal development world. Way back then he knew that failure was not a bad thing. He knew it was a stepping-stone towards something greater. He also knew that discouragement is part of this journey.

I may not have been taught this when I was growing up, but it's not too late now. I can tap through all of my disappointments and discouragement and find relief from the emotions tied around this.

As I tap, I see what Dale Carnegie meant, and how spot on he was. I get to allow myself to feel my way through my discouragement and disappointments and get to the other side.

I like knowing I can learn how to develop my personal definition of success and then move towards that without allowing discouragement to be the end of the line for me.

It's just a stepping-stone to success.

THOUGHT FOR THE DAY: *Discouragement and failure are just stepping-stones on my journey in life*

February 22

> *"Failure is the condiment that gives success its flavor."* —Truman Capote

When I'm done with these next few days, I suspect I will really have a new attitude towards failing. I may be stuck in different cycles of failing in my life, and yet I bet there's a silver lining in all of my failings.

There's a lot of truth to the idea that failure makes success taste better. It makes me realize that I can change and shift and need not stay stuck.

I bet if I talk to anyone who has been considered an overnight success, they might laugh or even roll their eyes and tell me their tales of how long their journey actually was to this "overnight success" they supposedly obtained.

Many things are taught in the culture I live in that I've likely bought into, but how could I not when I'm bombarded daily with messages about success from such a materialistic view?

Now is my chance to unhook from this programming and find my own unique journey and voice.

THOUGHT FOR THE DAY: *Seeing failure in a new way brings me relief and allows me to begin again.*

February 23

"You are allowed to be both a masterpiece and a work in progress simultaneously."

—Sophia Bush

What a novel idea in this fast-paced, you-better-have-your-shit-together world I live in.

I am definitely a work in progress. It's unlikely I'd still be in this body here on planet earth otherwise. Science says the universe is constantly expanding and changing, so why wouldn't I be as well?

When I settle into the idea that I will continue to be a work in progress and I am also born a masterpiece, I will find more peace of mind.

I might find I can laugh at myself more. I cannot take myself so freaking seriously. I can joke about my flaws and foibles. This is when I'm embracing my humanity.

I've heard that the beauty is in the imperfections, but who came up with what the actual imperfections are? If I think about it, the ideas of success, beauty, and more, are all products of a culture that has refined them again and again. It's all random.

Now I can embrace all parts of me. Tapping can help me to do this as I tap through the limits that got placed in my way over the years. I like that I can change my perspective around myself in this and begin to embrace myself more fully.

THOUGHT FOR THE DAY*: Today I can practice seeing the masterpiece I really am, a work in progress and all.*

February 24

"Focus on progress, not perfection."
—Unknown

When I pay attention to the little wins I experience every day, I see a different reality. My focus shifts from what's not working to what is working—to all the little shifts I'm making in the right direction. This builds momentum. I tune into what's going well, and the more I do this, the more I see a change for the better.

If I get tripped up and circle the drain with some less than desirably thoughts, I can be grateful that I'm catching myself in the act of this. That way, it doesn't matter how far down I've gone into the rabbit hole of negative self-talk. That I caught myself is the win because, when I do this, I'm interrupting the thought pattern and it changes it the more I do this. That's how I make lasting change. A little win is a big win.

I can be reminded again and again that I can't stop my thoughts, but I can interrupt them. Over time, this rewires my brain.

I'll see the evidence of these little wins. I notice that my resting thought rate has become far less negative. Then I notice my resting thought rate is firing off more positive and uplifting thoughts.

Progress, not perfection.

This is a key to creating lasting, positive change within me, which then reflects in my outside world.

THOUGHT FOR THE DAY: *Today I focus on my progress. My little wins*

February 25

"Every success story is a tale of constant adaptation, revision and change."

—Richard Branson

Once again, I am reminded that I can make little adaptations every day, little revisions that create real change. The beauty is it doesn't actually require a lot of time every day to create lasting change.

As I become more conscious of who's running my show (the bully, the wounded child, the healthy authentic self), and what part of me is telling me the things I'm hearing, I will catch myself, and in those moments where my thinking is setting me up to feel bad, I can tap (even briefly) and this will make little adaptations.

The result is I feel better, lighter, and freer. I'll take this any day of the week.

THOUGHT FOR THE DAY: Today I can make little adaptations in my thinking when needed.

February 26

---

*"You may live in the world as it is, but you can
still work to create the world as it should be."*
—*Michelle Obama*

This speaks to the world I live in and to the messages I hear daily that can make me forget the truth of my being. If I hear something repeated enough, I start to believe it, so what I have been hearing over and over again from the world I live in, that may not actually be my truth. Who says the world's view is right? Who says it's right for me?

The unhooking process from the world's view is a journey. It can be like pulling an IV of continuous programming out of my arm, only the IV has spread its beliefs to every part of my body and being.

The saying, "Don't believe everything you think," applies here. Just because I learned it—just because I've heard it over and over again—doesn't mean any of it is true.

I'm meant to find my own way through this lifetime, and as I unhook from the messages of the crazy world I'm living in, I become able to create the world as it should be for me.

THOUGHT FOR THE DAY: Today I will practice checking in and asking myself: what do I think? What do I feel?

February 27

"Love yourself first and everything else falls into line. You really have to love yourself to get anything done in this world."
—Lucille Ball

Learning to love myself is another journey I want to undertake in this life, but in a world that would have me think less of myself unless I fit into a certain mold, it can be challenging.

But I'm not alone on this journey. I can tune into God, the Universe, The Great Spirit, The Divine, The Dinosaurs, Fred Flintstone, The Wiser Self. Whatever works for me.

As I learn to reconnect with this spiritual part of me, guidance and direction can come in ways that help me to love myself a little more every day.

I'm meant to love myself and think well of myself. I may have been programmed to think otherwise, but these thought patterns can be changed the more I attend to and interrupt them. This is where tapping can help me as I tune into the less than loving programming I learned and release it from my energy system.

I find that I need not try to love myself. Self-love bubbles up from within me. The way it's always intended to be.

THOUGHT FOR THE DAY: Today I will practice finding things about myself that are lovable. If I can't, I can tap, so I clear the way for self-love to come through me.

February 28

"Nothing is impossible, the word itself says 'I'm possible.'" —Audrey Hepburn

---

This may feel so far from the truth for me. Maybe I've been mired down in "impossible." If I am, it's because I got messages repeated to me over and over again about my limits.

The world often teaches us to limit ourselves, and we can get a lot of conflicting messages while we're growing up.

For example, you might have heard something like, "Reach for the stars. The sky's the limit," and then, with that same breath, "Don't get your expectations up too high. You don't want to be disappointed." Or perhaps even, "No one has ever done that before. Be careful." These messages get into our psyche and our physiology and create limits and confusion within us.

Yet, as I unravel the craziness of the world I live in, I can see that there's so much more possible for me once I find relief and release from the limiting beliefs buried within me.

As I free myself from these limitations with tapping, I gain more access to the prefrontal cortex—the nonreactive, more creative, rationally thinking part of my brain. If I'm a spiritual person, I'm opening up to a Higher Power.

Either way, I can move beyond what has been limiting me to a place of possibility.

THOUGHT FOR THE DAY: Today I can try tapping when I hear the voice that says "impossible," just to find relief. In this way, I open up to more possibilities.

February 29

> *"You can start with nothing, and out of nothing and out of no way, a way will be made." ~Michael Bernard Beckwith*

In other words, more possibility. As I continue making the little shifts in my thinking with tapping, what I can find is that the clouds part, and the muck clears in my mind. When this happens, I have more experiences where things just come to me.

Someone calls me out of the blue with what I need. I overhear someone talking and there's an answer in what they are saying. I hear something on the radio that guides me to another piece of the puzzle unraveling in front of me.

I'm not having to push harder, work harder, or do better; it's as if just what I need keeps coming. I get an intuitive impulse I act on and things fall into place. It's a flow where things just keep coming and before I know it, I'm smiling brightly at how things are working out for me and not with a pushing, get it done energy.

Could it be I'm in the flow of life? And isn't this really the way it's meant to be for all of us? I just know I like it a lot.

THOUGHT FOR THE DAY*: What if today I can repeat to myself when things feel hard, "I'm open to the flow."*

March

March 1

---

*"Conformity is the jailer of freedom
and the enemy of growth." —John F.
Kennedy*

Living in the world I live in may have required my inner child to conform, to follow the rules, to color inside the lines to fit in. As a child I had to make sure that I did what was required of me and ensure that I stayed loyal to my tribe, my family, and those I was closest to.

What happened because of this is I unknowingly placed parentheses around my life. I learn to put limits on what was possible for me, particularly if my tribe didn't agree with my choices.

For example, I might have been the overachiever because that's what was expected of me, so I let go of my dream of being an artist. I might have been the responsible kid, so I put everyone else's needs ahead of my own and grew up too fast. I might have been the problem kid, who carried the family's secrets and angst. These were the silent contracts we all made with each other. I lost myself in the process and blamed myself for the plight of my life.

What if today I can begin again? I can use tapping to uncover my unconscious programming and free myself from the ties that bound me to a tribal loyalty that doesn't serve me anymore. I can know myself in a deeper, more genuine way and determine what calls me forward. I can take baby steps if necessary, so I feel good about what I'm doing and allow myself to adjust to this new way of being if I get scared.

It's never too late to begin again. Time will pass anyway. I can try it and do it, so it resonates with me. I might find freedom on the other side.

THOUGHT FOR THE DAY: *What if today I can do one simple thing that honors me? If I'm not even sure what that is, I could ask myself this: If I had to guess, what would be one thing I can do today to honor me? Then see if something pops in your head.*

March 2

> *"Self-compassion is simply giving the same kindness to ourselves that we would give to others."* — Christopher Gemer

When I judge myself, I'm lacking compassion for myself. I could judge myself for this. The other thing that judging myself does is it actually blocks me from real change.

When I judge myself, I actually lose the ability to create positive, lasting change. I might change something because I'm down on myself, but more often than not what follows is a "relapse," or my self-protecting mechanisms kick back in and my progress is lost.

I hear a lot about self-sabotaging behavior, but even the term self-sabotaging is by nature judgmental. The truth is anything I do that appears to not serve me is actually a way I protect myself. In the converse, anything I don't do that would actually help me is the opposite end of the same spectrum—it's still a form of self-protection. It's typically an unconscious form of self-protection, but it's still a way I'm attempting to protect myself.

When seen from this vantage point, I might be able to soften some of my self-judgment and actually have some compassion for why I do what I do.

If I struggle with self-compassion, I can tap on it and see what surfaces. As I clear some of the muck that's in my way, it's likely that I will find I become more compassionate towards myself. Self-compassion becomes a by-product of tapping through the ways I've learned to judge myself and thus lack compassion for myself.

THOUGHT FOR THE DAY: *What if today I can commit to noticing if I speak to myself in a way that lacks compassion? If I catch myself doing this, what if I can practice saying something compassionate, even if I don't believe it yet? It's still a way to practice.*

March 3

> *"I'm thankful for the challenges early on in my life because I have a perspective on the world." —America Ferrera*

As I heal from my past and the programming I adopted from the repetitive messages I've been exposed to, I do find that, with the benefit of hindsight, I now have a new perspective on my challenges early in life.

The veil gets lifted, and I'm able to see that what I went through has made me the person I am today. I can see that everything that came before now came to help me become exactly who I am now.

Challenges in life need not define me anymore. They are events that have happened that have shaped me into this amazing, wonderful human I am now—flaws, foibles, and all.

I'm this mixture of so many things, all of which can be honored because every single thing about me makes me the intricate person I am right here and now.

THOUGHT FOR THE DAY: *What if today I can lean into the idea that I am exactly as I am right now because of everything that has happened before today.*

March 4

"I have come to believe that caring for myself is not self-indulgent. Caring for myself is an act of survival." —Audre Lorde

I live in a world that teaches me to always put others before myself. If I don't, I might be self-indulgent or self-serving. However, if I ponder what caring for myself means, it means filling up my own cup first.

Doesn't it make sense that if I care for myself first, I will then have so much more to give? I'm no longer an empty well that's just running on pure adrenal from task to task.

"Just one more thing and then I'll chill out."

"Just one more thing and then I'll go to bed."

"Just one more thing and then I'll take that walk for myself."

"Just one more thing, and then I'll read that book."

In this face-paced world, I can easily one-more-thing myself into exhaustion. If I'm giving just because I think I should, no one benefits. This breeds resentment, irritation, and potential health challenges.

When I tap, I am clearing away the muck that has been in the way of me seeing I do matter. My needs are important, and as I learn to fill up my own cup, I replenish myself. When I do this, I have so much more space to give from the most genuine part of me, and this fills me up even more.

THOUGHT FOR THE DAY: *What if today I can open to the idea that caring for myself is imperative to living a more fulfilled life?*

March 5

"You may encounter many defeats, but you must not be defeated." —Maya Angelou

---

I don't want to stay stuck in feeling defeated, but how do I get to the other side of it? I may have learned all about overcoming obstacles, but there are times I just want to throw in the towel. Defeat has me in its grips, and it doesn't seem to let go.

I may hear many quotes about overcoming the odds and not staying in the pit of defeat, but has anyone ever shown me how to rise above it?

The personal development world might tell me to put on my big girl or big boy pants and just do it, whatever that means, but I want to know how to feel good and not feel like I'm pushing myself to cross some imaginary finish line that was never mine to begin with.

What if the how involves going into the feeling of defeat and exploring what's really beneath it? Tapping is a technique that can allow me to do just this. I might need the support of a skilled practitioner, but whatever I chose, I can use the defeat to unpack what's intensifying this for me. This can open me up to what limits have me in their grasp and as I explore and release the potent emotions attached to defeat, I can find liberation and freedom on the other side.

I can find that I'm now moving forward whereas in the past I may have stopped myself.

Going into the emotions also opens me up to guidance and direction that can help me once I have found relief from all the heavy thundering of emotions that yank me around if they're not allowed and released.

THOUGHT FOR THE DAY: *What if today I use tapping to help me find relief (if needed) around feeling defeated?*

March 6

"True life is lived when tiny changes occur." —Leo Tolstoy

What a relief to actually lean into the idea that life really is about incremental changes that can lead me to a more fulfilling life.

What if I already am the best version of myself? This isn't something I have to create within me because it's already there.

As I learn to deal with what's right in front of me in my emotional landscape, I can find relief from the patterns of thinking that I'm not enough, or I'm less than. These thoughts create potent emotions that make me believe these negative thoughts about myself.

I can be reminded that I am not the thoughts that I'm thinking. I'm the one witnessing the thoughts.

I am not my thoughts. Thoughts come and go. It's when my thoughts get tripped up, and I believe all kinds of crazy stories, that my thoughts feed me.

This is where simply interrupting my thoughts when I catch them has the power to set me free. As I keep interrupting them, I'll notice that the dark thoughts feel less and less true. This is evidence that I'm shifting my physiology and thus my resting thoughts rate becomes more optimistic because I'm no longer believing everything I'm thinking.

I'm witnessing the tiny shifts in my perception, and these little changes have the power to transform my life.

THOUGHT FOR THE DAY: *What a relief that a little change has the power to become a big change. What if today I can notice even one little change within me?*

March 7

"You alone are enough. You have nothing to prove to anybody." —Maya Angelou

---

Oh, if only I believed this. Yet what if I do believe this over time? What if as I tap through my beliefs around not being enough, or the need to explain myself or prove something to anyone, I find relief? When I find relief, I feel freer.

I might notice that someone disagrees with me and I can be okay with that without feeling the need to explain myself. I might notice that someone criticizes me, and it rolls off; I don't get attached to their criticism. I'm free when these moments happen.

I'll take more of these moments, please.

How do I get to these moments? I get to them by tapping when I find I am believing I'm not enough or I have something to prove. As I go into these learned limits, I uproot them, and they release their grip on me a little more each time I do. Over time, as my thoughts naturally become more positive, what I see outside of me becomes more positive.

If I remind myself that change happens in little increments, it's likely I'll stop putting so much pressure on myself to see fast results. I didn't believe these limits about myself overnight. They were imprinted with a lot of repetition, and this is actually a pathway to turning this around for me.

THOUGHT FOR THE DAY*: What if today I can find one moment to interrupt my thoughts around not feeling like I'm enough? What if that is enough for today?*

March 8

> *"If the path before you is clear, you're probably on someone else's." —Unknown*

This is interesting to ponder; let me do that right now. Maybe this idea that I could be on someone else's path includes having thoughts like, "I need to go to school, get a job, buy a home, and/or have a family," even when that doesn't actually feel right for me. Maybe I'm one of those people with my future mapped out for me by the society I live in.

What if this seems like the clear path I should take, but there's always been something else stirring inside of me that whispers about how there's something different out there for me?

Perhaps a different path reveals itself through the impulses I feel. For example, maybe some thought that's not even a thought tells me to pick up that phone and make that phone call, or to go left here instead of right. Maybe it tells me to grab that book that just fell off the shelf and see what it opened to, and so on. This alternative path seems a lot less clear because only small, seemingly inconsequential steps are being revealed here and there, and yet something still feels right.

Then, suddenly, the bully in my brain kicks in. It sends doubts through my head, and the path feels foggy, and now I feel afraid to consider so much as pursuing it further. But what if I got wired backwards in this world I grew up in? What if these little impulses are a byproduct of interrupting thoughts that aren't serving me? What if, by indulging these impulses, I am opening up to a new way of living and being? This new path may not always seem clear but, beyond the doubts the bully likes to lob my way, it feels right? It might be worth a try.

THOUGHT FOR THE DAY: *What if today I can see if I receive a little impulse to do something and act on it to see what happens?*

March 9

"Don't fear change. You may lose something good, but you may also gain something great." —Unknown

Easy for you to say, but what if I do fear change?

This is where tapping comes in. I need not put pressure on myself and tell myself that I shouldn't fear change. In fact, I can step into my fear of change and tap through it, so it finds a path out of my nervous system and thus out of me.

When this happens, I have effectively used the fear of change to release the fear of change. I go into it, I allow it, and I give it its airtime, and the amazing thing is the fear of change diminishes. I seem to magically be less afraid by embracing my fear of change instead of just telling myself I shouldn't fear it to begin with.

I like this way a lot. It's a great reminder that I can't stop my thoughts, but I can interrupt them. I can go into the thoughts and all the emotions they elicit in me, and freedom and liberation become my gifts as I move through my fear of change.

THOUGHT FOR THE DAY: *What if today I can remind myself that the way through my fears is to go into them with tapping so they can ultimately be released?*

March 10

"Do the best you can until you know better. Then when you know better, do better."

—Maya Angelou

I will know when I know to do better and not a moment before. If I'm still not "doing better," it's because I'm actually not ready yet, just like Maya Angelou is saying.

I might intellectually know better, but maybe I don't emotionally know better yet (i.e., in my head I might know better, but my heart isn't congruent with it yet), and this is okay; emotionally knowing better is the greater journey.

As I release more of the emotional blockages in my physiology, it frees up my emotional space and allows me to see things differently. In tapping, when someone gains a new perspective on an old problem, it's called a cognitive shift. On their own, they express seeing an old problem from a new vantage point. They have their "Ah-hah!" moment, where something they have been told finally feels true.

When this happens for me, I will do better, and it won't be because I pushed myself or bargained with myself to do better. I just do better because I want to. I'm now congruent with the changes needed and they happen with a lot more ease.

THOUGHT FOR THE DAY*: I will do better when my mind sees things differently and my emotions now have followed.*

March 11

"Change your thoughts and you change your world." —*Norman Vincent Peale*

Here's where the how comes up again. I believe that when my thoughts change, my outer world changes, and the "how" in how this happens can be answered with tapping (as one option).

When I catch myself circling the drain, elbow deep in dark thoughts, I can tap and go deeper into this way of thinking and ultimately find that the relief that's so important to my well-being.

Finding relief is all I have to reach for. Sometimes relief means I was in the pit of despair, but I have now moved onto feeling angry. This is a win if I can see it that way.

Despair has hopelessness within it. Anger can be both healthy and unhealthy, so when I've been debilitated with despair, and I'm now angry, I'm actually moving in the right direction. I don't intend to stay stuck in anger, but what if being angry instead of feeling despair is enough for me at this moment? Then, as I make my anger okay, I can eventually move to a better feeling place.

It's always good to remember that there's not a single bad or forbidden emotion; it's the actions that can come from the deeper suppression of emotions that can cause problems in my world.

As I learn to embrace all of my thoughts with tapping, I can find that my thoughts do change and become more uplifting naturally.

THOUGHT FOR THE DAY: *My thoughts are just thoughts. They need not define me anymore. They come and go and tapping helps to move them through me.*

March 12

---

*"You don't lead by hitting people over
the head - that's assault, not leadership."*
—Dwight D. Eisenhower

How often have I led myself in this way? How often have I unknowingly bullied myself? When I judge myself, I am essentially assaulting myself. When I make myself wrong for thinking my thoughts and feeling my feelings, I am hitting myself over the head.

The bully in my brain can get into my face with hideous thoughts that send me reeling. Thoughts that sound like:

"Who do you think you are?"

"You're a loser. Look at how well they're doing and look at you."

But the bully can also sound reasonable.

"You really should call your mother."

"Do you really need that second donut?"

However the bully in my brain might sound, it's an assault on myself. It's hitting myself over the head. This is not me leading me, this is me bullying me. If, however, I continue to notice when thoughts like this fire off in my mind, I can use tapping to interrupt them before they gain too much momentum.

Tapping has a cumulative effect, so as I tap to interrupt these thoughts, over time I will notice I am being more kind to myself. I'm leading myself towards remembering the authentic self I am below all the world's programming.

THOUGHT FOR THE DAY: *What if even one time today I can catch my inner bully in the act and interrupt it?*

March 13

"All great changes are preceded by chaos." —PictureQuotes.com

---

In the world I live in this seems to remain a truth, but what if I can go within to a place where I no longer have to use chaos to precede positive changes in my life?

What if, as I continue to release the muck that holds me back, I adjust along my path, much like a plane adjusts to stay on course so it can land? What if I make course corrections along my path that allow me to not have to be drenched in chaos to decide that change is needed?

If chaotic events do happen, what if I can now move through them with a lot more grace and ease? I allow myself all of my feelings, and I use tapping to move through these events so chaos can now be met with empowered transitioning. I move through life's events with more emotional intelligence as I've practiced being more emotional fit every day.

THOUGHT FOR THE DAY: *What if, in my world, I can learn that chaos no longer has to be the only fuel for positive lasting changes?*

March 14

"I'm on the hunt for who I've not yet become." —Unknown

Should I hunt for who I have yet to become? What if it's possible that, from a broader perspective, I already am who I'm meant to be?

Could this be the culture I live in that's talking? This culture pushes the ego's agenda, which says there is something missing in me, and I need to find it and fix it. What a relief it could be to entertain the idea that I need not fix myself because I already am exactly as I should be.

I'm in a human body, and along with this human experience comes a palette of amazing emotions I am meant to feel. Otherwise, why would I have them? Wouldn't it be helpful to believe that there's nothing I need to hunt for? That there's nothing I need to do or acquire or pursue?

If I just spend some time in quiet contemplation, staring at a sunset, watching the ocean, or taking in a mountain, doesn't this often create some feeling in me that is peaceful, or that just simply feels good? In these moments, I did nothing to create this feeling; the feeling just came from looking at something that can be awe-inspiring. What if these moments are moments where I'm actually tuning into the most authentic part of me? The part of me that need not do anything specific to feel good.

What if tapping is a tool I can use to clear away enough of the world's programming so I can have more of these moments?

THOUGHT FOR THE DAY*: What if today I can spend 3-5 minutes looking at something in nature and see what happens?*

March 15

"Work until your rivals become idols."
—Drake

I don't think I want this, do I? Do I want to spend this precious life working to make others idolize me? I live in a world that revere's famous people—the people who seem to "have it all." What if this is part of what haunts my mind and actually has me feeling bad about myself?

"I'm not like them."

"I don't have what they have."

"I'm not as successful as them."

Tapping can quell the voice of the bully in me that tells me I'm somehow less than because I'm measuring myself against some random societal standard that tells us all who we should be and what we should have.

I can begin to break-free from this madness?

This thinking only serves to have me feeling bad about myself, and I think I've had enough of that today.

THOUGHT FOR THE DAY*: What if today I can practice awakening to my not having to believe what the world or anyone else feeds me about who I am and what I should be doing with my life?*

March 16

"Smile at a stranger and you might change a life." —Steve Maraboli

---

What a concept that something so simple could carry such an impact.

I may have heard about something like this before. Stories of someone having an awful day and was feeling like life wasn't worth living, and then someone sent them the most amazing gift—a smile—and it was just what they needed. Something shifted in them, and they remembered that they were so much more than the crappy thoughts currently plaguing them. They lifted themselves above the crazy bully in their brain and remembered who they were at that moment. All because of a smile.

What if I can practice smiling at myself in the mirror and see what happens? What if it starts here within me? I smile at myself and give myself a gift.

What if this opens me to something so much better? I realize that I am the most important person in my life, and what if this spills out into the world to others?

Whatever way I want to try this—I start with smiling at others and move to myself, or the other way around—I bet something amazing might come from this. It might be worth a try.

THOUGHT FOR THE DAY: *What if I can practice smiling at myself today and see what happens?*

March 17

*"Actually, I just woke up one day and
decided I didn't want to feel like that
anymore, or ever again. So I changed. Just
like that." —curiano.com*

I may have had this experience at some point. It does happen. But what if this hasn't been my experience at all? What if I've been desperate to change something, and despite all my trying, I've only felt like I'm failing? Each time I try and seem to fail, my mood and how I perceive myself drops more.

What if this is the perfect place for tapping to enter, front and center? I get to tap through my self-judging talk and my trying and failing cycle and find relief. Not nirvana, just relief.

What if this is enough? I don't even have to pressure myself to tap because, even though tapping works well if you're consistent, what if simply honoring my unique journey has the bigger impact? It often seems like anything I genuinely let myself off the hook for creates breathing room for my true self to step in and take over. The healthy part of me takes the lead, and I act out of inspiration rather than the have to's and the shoulds.

I kinda like this idea a lot.

THOUGHT FOR THE DAY: *What if today I can let myself off the hook when I catch myself caught up in the have to's and the shoulds?*

March 18

---

*"One reason people resist change is
because they focus on what they have to give
up, instead of what they have to gain."*
—Rick Godwin

This can be true for me if I recognize that I'm resistant to change. If I'm someone who holds onto certainty, there's a good chance that I've dealt with a lot of uncertainty growing up, so it makes sense that the wounded child in me would grasp for certainty. The certainty seems to quell anxiety and fear.

The thing about my own evolution, though, is that what I grasp for eludes me. It's not that I've done anything wrong, or that I'm not aligning with my true heart's desires. I'm not being punished.

What if instead, from a soul perspective, my soul came here to expand? What if this expansion happens when I find myself in that interesting place of grasping and not receiving? What if I'm meant to learn how to let go of the death grip I needed to have growing up to survive? What if this is the pathway to true freedom?

I'm no longer haunted by what I don't have. I'm no longer afraid of what might happen. I slowly open to the idea that life has a way of working things out in a way that's far better than my wounded child or the bully in my brain thinks it ever could.

THOUGHT FOR THE DAY: *I like that this could be possible and I'm willing to open to this possibility, even just a little bit.*

March 19

"Every great and deep difficulty bears in itself its own solution. It forces us to change our thinking in order to find it." —Niels Bohr

---

In tapping, one of its coolest features is its ability to generate changes in my beliefs. This is called having a cognitive shift. The brain can see something from a new perspective, and this new perspective changes me on the inside.

When I get stuck in the difficulty of a problem, I don't have access to the less reactive, more creative, critical thinking part of my brain—the prefrontal cortex. However, when I tap on the problem, I release the energy that's been given to the problem. This lowers cortisol levels in my body. With less cortisol, also known as the stress hormone, my nervous system calms down and this gives me access to my less reactive, creative, critical thinking part of the brain that helps me generate solutions.

If I want to consider a spiritual side of things, I can virtually get the same results by setting the intention that, despite the difficulty, the perfect solution is already chosen. I need not believe this, but if I did believe this was possible, how differently might I feel?

Even if I don't believe this idea, does it feel at least a little better than the idea that I have a difficulty I can't find a solution to?

Whether I follow the way of science or the way of spirituality, the results are the same. To find that solutions come either from a calmer mind, a Higher Power or both, is noteworthy.

THOUGHT FOR THE DAY*: What if today I can consider that there is a solution to any problem, and finding relief from my spinning thoughts is a great place to start?*

March 20

"The secret of change is to focus all of your energy, not on fighting the old, but on building the new." —Socrates

This is a spin off from yesterday's reading, only maybe this is being said in a different way that helps me. When I'm in fight mode, I have no space for anything else. Fighting begets more fighting. Here's another way for me to look at what Socrates is saying:

I need not focus all of my energy on building something new. I can't if I have a lot of build up from trying to fight the old. As soon as I go deeper into the fight with tapping, it shifts. It relieves. The benefit of this is that I will find I naturally focus on the new.

When tapping started, tapping through the negative was the primary focus, and people got better. Why would this be? What if people got better because what they were doing by tapping through the negative was removing the learned limits that got placed on them? What if this allowed the space for who they are—a limitless, infinite being—to come to the forefront in their lives?

What if the same is true for me?

THOUGHT FOR THE DAY: *What if today I can open to the idea that within me is a limitless, infinite being?*

March 21

"Change brings opportunity."
—Unknown

Once again back to change, but it is true. Whether I like it or not, change is the one thing I can depend on.

It might take time for change to be seen, but things are always changing. My physiology is always changing. Nature is always changing. Nothing is static. Change might move at a pace where it's easy to miss the daily changes..

When something happens in my life that causes a change I feel resistant to, it's hard (if not impossible) to see there can be new opportunities for me because of it.

My physiology can get in the way. When I'm feeling stressed because I'm afraid or uncertain, and things feel daunting, I can't see the opportunities being created. When I tap, I soothe my physiology and my emotional landscape, and from this soothed place I now can see what's possible, and the opportunities. This happens as I honor my truth with tapping and allow the potent emotions and fearful thoughts to be attended to.

THOUGHT FOR THE DAY*: What if today is a day I can tap if I feel stressed about some potential change? That's all I have to do. This allows for what needs to come to come.*

March 22

"I can't change the world, but I can change the world in me." —Bono

---

What if I do change a lot of things I touch in this world as I change the world within me?

I don't change the world within me with an agenda about what needs to come because of my inner work. I do it because I want peace more than anything. Pushing for change hasn't worked out that well for me.

While I may have seen results from the "fruits of my labor," or the pushing the world teaches, what if it's a different experience if I'm attending to my inner world because I want peace for me? I'm not attached to a particular outcome. I might prefer it, but I'm free because I need not have it a certain way. I'm free because I'm open to allowing something greater to come. I'm learning to trust I need not have all the answers or figure it all out.

As I learn to let go of particular outcomes, I'm allowing for things to work out even better, in ways that might just pleasantly surprise me. What a much easier way to live. Tapping is my tool to help me release what's keeping me from this experience. It helps me deal with my humanness so I can experience the most amazing aspects within me.

THOUGHT FOR THE DAY: What if today I can check my intentions for desiring change? If I find I have an agenda, that's okay. I can note this and ask to be relieved of my agenda.

March 23

"Your soul is the power and core of
who you are. Feed it well." —Anonymous

The world I live in feeds my ego self. It feeds the bully and the wounded child part of my ego. When these parts of me run my show, they drowned out my soul. It's good to know that just because the voice inside of me is loud and demanding doesn't mean that it's the true me talking. If it is loud and demanding, it's not the true me.

The voice of the outside world is a doer extraordinaire; it's impatient and likes to push for things to happen. The true me speaks quietly and lovingly. It's not demeaning or demanding. It never tells me to put my big girl or big boy pants on. It talks the way a loving parent or mentor would. It sends me sweet little messages that direct me to the single next step for me.

The more I tap, the more I can find that my true self takes over and guides my steps.

THOUGHT FOR THE DAY: I realize I don't have to figure anything out. I get the guidance and steps I need from within.

March 24

"Today I have the power to change my story." —Unknown

Tapping clears the way for me to change my story. My story can change because of the tapping. The shifts in perspective it can bring change my story without me trying to change it.

As I keep honoring all of my feelings, and as I find more relief from the learned limits I unknowingly adopted, my story unfolds independent of any agenda and my life comes through me in amazing ways. This happens because my true self is now the one guiding me through this journey called life.

THOUGHT FOR THE DAY: *As I tap through the limiting story I've learned to see as my "truth," these self-imposed limits dissipate, and my outlook becomes more positive without me really trying.*

March 25

"Happiness is not a goal. It's a by-product of a life well lived." —Eleanor Roosevelt

When I make happiness a goal, there's a good chance I'll miss feeling it. Happiness is a feeling. It's an experience. The things I do to create happiness are just things.

If I watch an animal playing, I bet if I tune in, it's likely I'm feeling happy. If I spend time petting my cat or dog, I bet I feel happy. If I spend time with my children and I'm present and engaged with them, I bet I feel happy. In cases like these, happiness is a by-product of making choices that feel good.

I can think of many times where my mouth said yes to something that my heart said no to. If I notice this pattern with some detachment, and tap to find relief, the more I practice this over time, the more I'll say no when it's a no for me.

THOUGHT FOR THE DAY*: What if today I can consider that sometimes saying yes to me means saying no to someone else?*

March 26

"Be a good person, but don't waste time to prove it." —e.Buddihism.com

---

Good people don't tell you how good they are, they just are. This is the humility they have that is so endearing. I want to do good for no other reason than it feels good. If I see I have an agenda behind doing good, or I expect getting something in return, then I'm not clean about it.

Even if I'm trying to be a good person so I can reach salvation of some sort, that's an agenda. I do this so I can get this in return.

When my heart calls me forward to help someone, or to smile at a stranger, or to give words of encouragement, and I act, I'm coming from a place of inspiration.

Forcing or pushing myself to "do good things" when I don't want to doesn't make me a bad person, and it doesn't make me wrong. It just makes me human. As I learn to honor my humanity, sometimes saying yes to myself means saying no to someone else. This is so important because I am far more able to give cleanly when I'm meeting my own needs. The world I live in often teaches the opposite. Bend over backwards for everyone else. Put yourself last. Even sayings like, "I can sleep when I'm dead," is actually self-punishing because that's the bully talking in a way that's clever. It can sound like motivation, but it's not me being kind to myself, the most important person in my life.

THOUGHT FOR THE DAY*: What if today I can find one simple way to be kind to myself? This is a great place to start.*

March 27

> *"What you aim at determines what you see." —Jordan Peterson*

There's a lot of truth in this, however there's a big "but" here. When I've grown up not learning how to be good, kind, or loving to myself, my aim is focused on what I learned: scarcity, fear, anxiousness, loss, lack of trust, and so much more.

It's also likely that I received a lot of mixed signals. Things from, "The skies the limit," to, "Oh, that's just setting yourself up for failure."

If I grew up with mixed signals (or messages that were less than desirable, shall I say), what if my aim right now can be to go into my learned limits and use tapping to find relief, and then release from these learned limits?

If I tell myself I need to aim high, but my internal programming isn't congruent with this, guess what's going to happen? I will miss the mark, and not because I'm not capable. I'll miss the mark because I'm bumping up against the learned limits in my way.

As I home in on these learned limits and aim to release them, I find relief. I find I can move forward so it allows me to move past my learned limits instead of bumping into them and stalling out.

This is a different way to see my limitations. Hallelujah!

THOUGHT FOR THE DAY: *With tapping, I aim at my learned limits so I can release them.*

March 28

"Change… a gift disguised as discomfort." —Unknown

In the world I live in, change often gets a bad—if not confusing—rap.

I'm being told to embrace change, and yet if the change I experienced growing up was wrapped in anger and resentment, or based on traumatic experiences, change will definitely not feel like my friend now.

But I can rewrite my experiences around change with tapping. I can go into the events I remember that caused harm to my psyche and tap through them so I unhook from the discomfort that change can have.

As I do this, change becomes less of a challenge for me. I might even find I look forward to change, and maybe even get excited about it.

THOUGHT FOR THE DAY*: What if today I can weigh in on how I feel about change and tap if I need to, to find relief?*

March 29

"Small changes eventually add up to huge results." —Unknown

I don't think I can be reminded of this enough, especially in this fast-paced, make-it-happen world. A world that honors the ego, the superstars, the elite, and the go-getters. Learning to unhook from this craziness takes baby steps, especially considering how bombarded I am daily with all this madness.

There is a way out of this madness. An example would be I notice someone being revered who appears to "have it all" and I remind myself I'm not competing anymore.

The evidence of my unhooking shows up as I notice I'm not so triggered by someone else's success. This lets me know my physiology is changing and thus changing what's possible for me.

I'm learning to be true to myself and my journey each day. Small changes like this, over time, add up to huge results for me.

THOUGHT FOR THE DAY: *I walk my own unique path in this life.*

March 30

> *"All great achievements require time."*
> —*Maya Angelou*

This is another great reminder that, wherever I am in life, I'm doing good. I'm walking my own path, in my own way, learning to honor the amazing human that I am, independent of the craziness of the world around me.

What can help me remain true to me is catching that bully voice when it's feeding me the shit show. That voice tells me everything that's wrong. It's the voice that tells me that everything is bad or not going to work. It's the voice of constant comparison. It tells me that I'm less than them, but maybe better than those people. None of this feels good. I'm either one up or two down. When I'm in comparison mode, it's an indication the bully in my brain is running my show.

Through my awareness of this, I can interrupt this pattern of thinking and relinquish the unconscious hold this tyrant has on me. As I practice doing this, I find emotional freedom. This allows me to trust my unique path as I continue unhooking from the world's programming and agenda.

THOUGHT FOR THE DAY: *If I find myself comparing today, I can interrupt this pattern. This is me stepping forward to honoring me.*

March 31

> *"Sometimes you just need to go off the grid and get your soul right." —Charlene Whitman*

Being busy doesn't allow me the space to be present with my inner world. My soul is always available it just appears to have gone dormant because the voice of the busy world is so freaking loud.

I need not go on a retreat to reconnect with this part of me, but what if I can start with 3-5 minutes of sitting quietly every day, in nature, doing absolutely nothing except being present for a change. If I do this consistently, I might hear the whispers my soul sends. Those intuitive impulses that actually carry guidance and direction for my life's unfolding.

Actions get taken from a place of inspiration rather than the pushing of the world. My life unfolds without a list of goals I need to accomplish. My heart opens to greater awareness. I smile more. I might even find I'm living a more fulfilling version of my life, and I realize that I'm reconnecting with my soul.

I like this idea a lot. It feels soothing.

THOUGHT FOR THE DAY: *What if today I can give my soul 3-5 minutes off grid time?*

April

April 1

---

*"No one can make you feel inferior
without your consent." —Eleanore
Roosevelt*

As much as I might intellectually believe there is a great truth in this saying, I've spent a lot of time feeling inferior and having that mirrored back by those around me.

This has been my reality. If you don't grow up being reinforced about all the amazing qualities you have, you will hit some bumps in the self-esteem road.

I may have had awesome parents, but the bombardment of society's programming is enough to make even the most confident person question themselves. On top of which, just being human lends itself to times where I can feel inferior. The key is to learn to accept that I have a part of me that can get activated when I've been made to feel inferior. Who doesn't? It's part of being human.

What I can do when I notice that my inferiority issues are being triggered is I can go into the feelings that surface when I'm feeling inferior and tap through them. This allows my emotions to soften about this issue. The more I practice this when I get provoked, the more I'll find I feel less inferior when these situations arise.

The day will come when someone might be attempting to criticize or judge me, and I realize that it just rolls off of me. I don't attach to what they're saying about me. I don't personalize it.

This is a very different experience than someone simply telling me not to take it personally. That has never helped me. It takes repetitive practice to help me not take things personally. It's not as though I can command myself to stop taking things personally. As I go into the feelings that arise, how they land for me softens. This takes practice. This practice allows me to take things less personally less often over time.

THOUGHT FOR THE DAY*: What if today I can ask myself the following question? When I do take things personally, I do so because...*

Once I see what answer surfaces, this becomes my roadmap on where I should start tapping.

April 2

> *"It takes a special kind of mind to break away from the norm, to know or to believe that what everybody accepts is not right."*
> —*Wangari Maathai*

When I question my thoughts and what's been taught I can feel uncomfortable. The culture I live in has many things it says are right and wrong, good and bad, up and down, and on and on.

What if things get shaken up for me? I realize that many things I've been told aren't true, even if the majority of people agree.

Standards of beauty are programmed. Look at fashion magazines and advertising, for example. When I look at them, I'm seeing images repeatedly until the standards they set are what makes someone attractive.

Living a successful life is programmed through lifestyle marketing. If you drive this car, live in this house or neighborhood, have a certain job or business, you are succeeding according to cultural programming.

Each religion does this when they teach about their version of God. If I do this I'm a good person. If I do that, I'm a bad person. These are the things I need to do to be worthy (as if I'm not already inherently worthy).

I can pick any topic and find a cultural programming behind it.

To break away from societal norms can take vigilance. My mind gets bombarded every day with programmed messages meant to get me to buy something, or to be something, or to have something. This programming tells me my life will be much fuller if I have this or that.

Catching this programming takes my awareness of and presence to the messages I'm allowing in and believing. As my mind starts to break-free, I become more inquisitive. I reach this place where I wake up to all the programming, and my mind sees things differently. I see things differently from how I have seen them before. This has the power to change my life for the better.

THOUGHT FOR THE DAY: *What if I'm open to breaking away from the norms I've been taught? I like this idea a lot, and I'm open to seeing where this takes me.*

April 3

"Don't be defined by someone else's standards, have your own definition of success." —Duke Matlock

---

This thought goes hand in hand with yesterday's topic. It's hard not to compare myself with others. The culture I live in promotes competition over cooperation.

This is exactly why, as I wake up from the crazy programming I've been subjected to for many years, I realize that I can decide what success means. The more I continue to unhook from what the outside world tells me, the more I decide for myself what living a successful life means. My definition comes from within me; it's not measured by the world's standards anymore.

I wake up to just how insane all the pushing and driving is.

It's no wonder you hear famous people, who seem to have it all, talk about how empty having it all can be. How having it all is not where it's at, at all.

It's no wonder you hear about famous people who take their own life. They've reached what appears to be the pinnacle of success and feel lost and empty. They are still facing their own inner demons. The bully in their brain is still battling it out with their wounded inner child. Their coping mechanism may have been running from themselves through the busyness of success. This is a product of the culture I live in. Push harder, try harder, do more, succeed more. There's not space in this to go within and hear the authentic self speaking. How could they? It's not what the culture teaches.

That's why it's important for me to learn to open my mind to what's important to me, and not what the world tells me. I do this as I pay attention to my thoughts and question the validity of them.

THOUGHT FOR THE DAY: *What if today I can pay attention to my thinking for 3-5 minutes and practice noticing who's running my show: the bully, the wounded child, or my authentic self?*

April 4

"A life directed chiefly toward the fulfillment of personal desires will sooner or later always lead to bitter disappointment."
—Albert Einstein

If I pay attention to the world I live in, this is often what the world preaches. I may have heard the term New Cage, which is a clever spin on the New Age movement.

Humans created the New Age movement, along with all religions. This can boggle the mind when I awaken to these ideas.

Many religions, along with the New Age movement and the personal development world, teach how I have to follow a specific dogma and/or guidelines to be worthy of creating a fulfilling life. A worthwhile life. The Law of Attraction teaches that it's up to me to align myself with my desires so I can attract my heart's desires to me.

But what happens when my heart's desires don't come into being? If I'm honest with myself, I'll bet I feel bad. I'll bet I blame myself. I'll bet I go down the rabbit hole of asking what's wrong with me they can have their hearts' desires, but I can't. Whether it's religion, The New Age movement, The Law of Attraction, The Personal Development world, or any other institution that teaches exclusivity or has a lot of rules and dogma that need to be followed, these are all ego driven institutions.

This might just blow my mind a little bit, or maybe a lot, but they all have the power to make me judge and feel bad about myself if I'm not doing it right. All have the power to leave me way too hooked into pushing the ego's agenda. All have the power to lead me to a bitter and disappointing assessment of myself.

Am I meant to follow a list of tasks or behaviors in this lifetime? Or am I meant to open up to the truth of my being? If I accepted every part of me, wouldn't I approve of myself more? Wouldn't this actually promote self-love? Aren't I meant to see the best in myself?

THOUGHT FOR THE DAY: *What if learning to accept and love myself more each day actually leads me to a life where I am of service for the highest good for all whose lives I touch?*

April 5

"Personal development is not for broken people. It's for people who want a better life."

—Dave Hollis

If ever there was a quote about exclusivity, it's this one. It's literally telling me if I have broken parts of myself—which are the wounded parts of me—then I should not bother even dipping my toe in the personal development world.

Martin Luther King, Jr. preached inclusivity. He, too, was excluded and yet spoke of inclusivity for all. He referred to The Constitution of the United States when he said. "I have a dream that one day this nation will rise up, live out the true meaning of its creed: 'We hold these truths to be self-evident, that all men are created equal.'"

Are some of us actually created to be better than others? Am I better or less than someone else? When I ponder this, I think I can see the craziness of exclusivity. It wakes me up to how inclusivity just makes sense.

Tapping actually has the power to assist me in going into my wounding and find relief along with self-acceptance. As I become freer from my wounding, by going deeper into it, I do live a better life because I'm no longer being exclusive with myself and denying anything about myself. Emotional freedom becomes something I experience more and more. This also opens me up to the most authentic part of me, also called The Great Self.

THOUGHT FOR THE DAY: *Don't we all have a great self within us? What if I can tune into mine today, even if just for a moment?*

April 6

> *"You cannot dream yourself into a character; you must hammer and forge yourself one."*
>
> —*Henry David Thoreau*

Am I about to disagree with Henry David Thoreau? Let me think. Yes. Yes, I am. Here's another doozy of a quote I might want to question the validity of.

In the world I live in, this idea that I have to try harder, push more, and hammer myself into submission so I can create the life I want is what is often taught to us growing up.

This sounds exhausting. I think that when he wrote this quote, he was listening to the ego-based self. The bully in his brain had a fierce grip on him at that moment.

I know plenty of hard-working folks who have attempted to hammer themselves into submission to some randomly chosen perspective of what makes someone a worthwhile human. I want to escape from being a prisoner in this jail.

Tapping is such a beautiful process because it allows me the full and unadulterated truth of where I'm at in any moment. If I'm telling myself I need to hammer myself into a character, I can use tapping to explore this idea and see what learned limits are lurking below the surface in my psyche.

As I do this, I actually have a prison break from the ego's agenda. When this happens, it's likely that I become open to the guidance and direction that comes through me for the highest expression of this life. The amazing thing about this is that my life unfolds in amazing ways. I'm no longer the goal seeker. I'm the vehicle being used to express the highest in this life, and this includes all whose lives I touch.

If I check in, I realize there's no hammering necessary. Things just have a way of flowing with grace and ease.

THOUGHT FOR THE DAY: *What can I do today that feels light and easy?*

April 7

"You are essentially who you create yourself to be and all that occurs in your life is the result of your own making."
—Stephen Richards

Stick a fork in me, I'm done with this type of self-blame. This is what the world I live in teaches me: how to blame myself for everything that happens in my life.

What's missing in the personal development mumbo-jumbo is my soul.

What if many things that happen in my life are not happening because, once again, I've done something wrong? Once again, I'm not aligning properly with my desires. Once again, I'm not trying hard enough, or doing enough.

What if I came into this lifetime to evolve through circumstances that challenge me? What a nicer, kinder way to see things that happen in life.

I know plenty of people who work hard on themselves and still things don't seem to work out. If hard work got me what I wanted, I'd already have everything my heart desires, and then some, so there has to be something else going on here. The only thing that makes true sense is there are things that happen in my life to assist my evolution.

I've spent a lifetime blaming myself because that's what the world I live in tells me.

I want to unhook from this madness and find what's true for me, independent of the ego-based world I live in.

THOUGHT FOR THE DAY: *What if today I can tell myself that my life is unfolding for the sake of my evolution? I'm not meant to keep blaming myself. There's a force at work here that knows what it's doing.*

April 8

"Grow through what you go through."
—*SoloQuotes.com*

Yes. This is a great follow-up from yesterday. Instead of thinking that the things happening to me are my fault and are because I'm doing something wrong, I like this idea that things happen for my growth and evolution. What a relief.

I can hang up my brow-beating mantras and cut myself some slack. I can let myself off the proverbial hook and begin to be kinder to myself.

From this place, I see life differently. Life unfolds through me rather than me perpetually pushing the egos agenda. I become a vehicle for the highest for all, myself included.

I might be able to release the belief in a punitive, punishing God up in the sky messing with me. This type of being is an extreme narcissist, and at worse it's a psychopathic entity. I like the idea a lot that there's an entirely different way to see this.

What if each day I ponder a new outlook my life opens up to new possibilities so much greater than my human self can imagine? I get to shed the cloak of deception that's been shrouding a greater truth for me.

THOUGHT FOR THE DAY: *What if today I can ask to be used for the highest, then just see what unfolds?*

April 9

> *"Be patient with yourself. Self-growth is tender; It's holy ground. There's no greater investment." —Stephen Covey*

How lovely to be permitted to be tender with myself. I like this a lot. It's not something that's taught in our put-your-big-girl-or-boy-pants-on world.

What I can start doing is asking myself, "Who do I want to listen to today? Do I want to listen to the voice that punishes me, or do I want to listen to the voice that supports and uplifts me?"

I think I know my choice.

Then I can notice which voice is activated in me. It's not a 24/7 job. Most of the time, especially in the beginning, I won't notice who is talking. But when I do, these are precious moments. These are moments when my unconscious programming becomes conscious.

As I become more aware of my inner world, I interrupt the programming firing off on all cylinders. Over time, the bully in my brain gets quieter, and the authentic, healthy part of me becomes more prevalent. My thoughts become better for me over time, and my life becomes better. I become that ever evolving being I'm intended to be.

THOUGHT FOR THE DAY: *What if today I can set the intention to practice some patience and tenderness towards myself?*

April 10

"Don't compare your life to others.
There's no comparison between the sun and
the moon, they shine when it's their time."
—Unknown

To think that we all have our own growing and blooming seasons. What if I can remind myself that my growth and bloom cycle is unique?

When I find myself comparing I can repeat this mantra to myself:

My life is unfolding as it's meant to for me.

Comparing is always a losing battle, and yet it's so prevalent in the world I live in. I'm taught about winners and losers from the get-go. What if now is my time to unhook from the idea of winners and losers and just remind myself that we all have our own unique journey filled with whatever we need to evolve?

The more I unhook from a culture that teaches about winning and losing, the more I find my own path and my own awakening. I like this idea a lot.

THOUGHT FOR THE DAY*: I have my own unique growth and bloom cycle.*

April 11

"When you recall that only your thoughts can hold you hostage, you will be free from other people's judgments of you."
—Unknown

My thoughts can hold me hostage, but just being aware of this might not be enough to help me to find relief from this. Tapping is a highly effective way to go into the thoughts I carry around that are holding me hostage. As I tap through them, I find relief from the chokehold they have on me.

I become an observer of my thoughts. This helps me to separate myself from them. As I separate from them, I have more of a choice about which thoughts I will believe or agree with, and which thoughts don't serve my well-being. I can then discard the thoughts that don't serve me the more I practice separating from them.

I do this by asking myself, "Who is running my show right now? The bully or the wounded child?"

Once I learn who's in charge, this alone serves as an interruption of these thoughts and gives me the space to put my healthy adult self back into the driver's seat. The more I do this, the easier it gets, and the more emotionally fit I become.

THOUGHT FOR THE DAY*: If I find myself upset today or feeling badly, I can pause and ask myself, "Who's running my show right now?" This is a great beginning.*

April 12

"Remember, most of your stress comes from the way you respond, not the way life is. Adjust your attitude, and all that extra stress is gone." —best quotes.name

---

No kidding! Only I'd say that there's a big difference between responding and reacting.

Responding comes from a place of thoughtful consideration. Reacting is a loaded emotional hijack that takes me over. Maybe I already understand this. Maybe I don't. Either way, I don't want to react to people, so it hurts me or them.

When I'm feeling hurt by someone else's words or actions, I might feel like I want to hurt them back. I might not know this is operating in me, or I might know it and yet still be unable to stop myself from reacting. This is where tapping comes in. It's easy to tell myself that I need an attitude adjustment, but actually adjusting my attitude from reacting to responding takes practice.

It's likely I have some hardwired programming that sends me from zero to sixty quickly. Catching this is the first step and using tapping to tap through what's below my reactions is an important combination to effect positive, lasting change.

There's also a big difference between knowing something intellectually and knowing someone emotionally. As I tap through my reacting, I am doing the best thing I can to adjust my attitude because my attitude becomes adjusted with a lot more ease this way.

THOUGHT FOR THE DAY: *What if today I can tap if I find myself in reaction mode? Even if it's well after the fact.*

April 13

"Give your best every day." —Unknown

What if I can remind myself that, no matter how I behave or what I do, I am always doing the best I can every day? Therefore, I am giving my best every day, always. If in any moment of my life, I could do something differently or better, I would.

The most compassionate thing I can do for myself is to remind myself often that I am always doing the best I can at every moment. This is also true of everyone else I encounter. As I learn to give myself the benefit of the doubt, I ease up on myself and I begin to speak to myself, so it promotes and supports my well-being. The benefit of this is that my behavior becomes better for me because I'm being better to me. Internal changes create external changes in myself and with a lot more ease.

A way to promote this is to talk to my wounded inner child like I would talk to a child I wanted to help or, if I'm an animal lover, the way I talk to my dog or cat, or any animal I love and care for.

THOUGHT FOR THE DAY: *Let it begin with me.*

April 14

"An empty lantern provides no light.
Self-care is the fuel that allows your light to
shine brightly." —developgoodhabits.com

This is a great analogy, and yet I might have minimal skills when it comes to how I can practice self-care. Where do I even begin?

What if self-care is pausing when someone asks me to do something for them and weighing in on if I would agree out of guilt or out of a genuine desire to help? What if self-care is taking a moment to watch a bird, the sunset, notice a flower, pet an animal, smile at a stranger, or smile at myself in the mirror? What if this is a great beginning?

Otherwise, self-care may never happen in this fast-paced, get-er-done world I live in.

What if I can carve out little moments of self-care throughout my day, just to start? Even if it's just one moment a day. If I try this, I might find that I'm more likely to do a little more, and then maybe even a little more.

THOUGHT FOR THE DAY: *What if self-care can happen with little changes and be more lasting?*

April 15

"The truest success is but the development of self." —Charles Atlas

What if there's an even more beautiful combination here?

1) My willingness to deal with my humanness and find relief from the things that trip me up.
2) My willingness to practice turning things over to the God of my understanding when things don't appear to work out for me.

Being a human means I can try and take this course or do that program, and then if something I desire to be different isn't happening, then I can

126

consider that it's not meant to... yet. And then maybe it's not meant to be, ever, because there's something even better for me lining up. What a concept!

This idea can take so much of the worldly pressure off of me needing to make it happen or me needing to figure it out.

I like the idea that if somethings not happening that's on my list of goals or desires, a force at work in my life knows what it's doing and is actually guiding and directing me to something even better.

THOUGHT FOR THE DAY: *What if today I can remind myself that things could be working out for me regardless of appearance or the current state of affairs?*

April 16

> *"May your character preach more loudly than your words." —Mohamed Ayyed*

Anyone can say anything, but what someone does tells you who they are.

If I've been on this planet for any length of time, it's likely that I've had people tell me they would do something or change something, etc., and yet when it came down to it, zero, zippo, nada. Their actions speak their truth. This shows their (current) character.

Same is true for me.

If I continue to feel frustrated because someone I know keeps telling me they will do something and they don't, I can use tapping to go within and see what's going on. Not in a self-blaming way, but in a way where I'm seeking my own liberation.

As I uncover what's happening for me and tap through this, I can find liberation for me. This creates different behaviors within me. I find solutions that work for me.

The irony is that as I unhook from the other person and release the expectation, they can be something they're not, they show up differently. I let go of my agenda around them. Suddenly, they do the very thing I wanted them to do because I've detached.

As I've relaxed my own agenda around how things should be, things get resolved one way or another for me with a lot less angst. This allows me to display my character with my own actions rather than my words.

THOUGHT FOR THE DAY*: What if today I can value my character more than anything else?*

April 17

"Sometimes the people around you won't understand your journey. They don't need to, it's not for them." —The Good Quote

I may have learned to seek a lot of affirmation outside of myself. I seek the approval of others. This imprisons me, often without me realizing just how imprisoning it is.

When I expect anyone to differ from who they are, I feel frustrated and victimized when they aren't. There's a lot of talk that floats around about the victim mentality that makes it very challenging to admit I have a victim within me. Everyone does, so I have a lot of company. The challenge is that there's little acceptance around being the victim.

I live in a culture that victim blames all the time, so it could be very challenging for me to acknowledge and eventually honor the victim (in other words, the wounded child) within me.

When I was a child, I was a victim. It's highly unlikely that I could get away or remove myself from the crazy town I may have been a part of. I was too young and dependent on those around me to help myself. Maybe I wasn't helped, so I had to figure things out for myself. Children are actually brilliant in how they figure out how to adapt and survive their circumstances without outside help. As I start to see how brilliant my own wounded child (my inner victim) was, I might judge this part of me a whole lot less and learn to accept and maybe even love this part of me more. This learning to love and accept all parts of me is a pathway to inner freedom and emotional fitness.

As I do this, I'm less likely to look to others to understand me because I'm understanding myself. Ironically, I experience more understanding from others because I'm now detached from this need. I'm filling myself up from within.

THOUGHT FOR THE DAY: *What if today I can practice approving of myself in some small way?*

April 18

"Never give up on something that you really want. It's difficult to wait, but more difficult to regret." —Unknown

---

This is great in theory, but it can be hard in practice. Here's the thing I want to understand about myself: Do I have a death grip of sorts on something that I want? Am I grasping for it with angst? If I can feel peace about whether what I want comes to me or not, I'm free.

How do I do this? I practice turning over my desire to my version of a higher power. If I don't trust my version of a higher power, I can start by updating how I see my higher power. As I learn to update whatever could be a source of peace for me, it's easier to let go of my need for my desires to be fulfilled. This is a very different place to be because it's not me pushing the egos agenda; it's me learning to tune into a force of goodness that can guide and direct me for the highest good.

It could be possible that what I think I want and need isn't actually for my highest good. As I learn to soften the grip I have on my desires, I open up to something even better for me to come into my experience. This is a journey of unhooking from the world's agenda, the egos agenda.

The more I practice turning my desires over to a higher power, the more I open to the highest expression of things in my life, and the more amazing things can turn out with grace and ease.

THOUGHT FOR THE DAY: *What if today, if I notice I'm gripping onto some desire, I can practice turning it over to a higher power. I could say, "Take this from me. Show me how to let go and let you in."*

April 19

"There's a difference between giving up and knowing when you've had enough."

—Unknown

Absolutely! There's so much momentum around maintaining a death grip on something I believe is best for me. There's even a lot of shame preached around the idea that winners keep going while losers give up.

What if there's a different way to see this? What if, like this quote says, I've been holding on tightly to what I believe is best for me and it's still not happening? What if it's not happening, not because I'm doing it wrong or not trying hard enough, but because I'm meant to let go and allow the true self to take over and lead the way to a far better outcome for the highest and best for myself and all who are involved?

What if the big difference between giving up and knowing when it's time to let go is I move from ego-consciousness to higher-consciousness? I stop all the pushing the ego has me doing and open up to my soul taking over and guiding me to what's best.

What a difference!

THOUGHT FOR THE DAY: *What if today I can let myself know that it's okay to let go, even just a little bit, and allow my soul to guide me to what's best for me?*

April 20

"It's often the deepest pain which empowers you to grow into your highest self." —PictureQuotes.com

---

As a human this is often true. It's not because I'm doing anything wrong, it's just because that's the set-up in the world I live in.

The world loves stories about overcoming obstacles. Stories about how, against all odds, things turned around for someone. The down on their luck stories sell, probably because so many people have learned how to feel down and out in this world and these stories say there's hope it won't stay this way.

What if it could be possible that I need not be down and out to grow? It's not wrong I do it this way because that idea is taught in this world, but what if, as I learn to shift this paradigm in myself, I find that things get better?

It doesn't mean I have to practice spiritual bypass at all (e.g., just think happy thoughts and it will all be okay). It means I honor all of my emotions and all parts of me, but I learn to rewrite the down and out story for myself so I can learn and grow in the best of circumstances as well and allow more of this into my life.

Something to consider.

THOUGHT FOR THE DAY*: What if today I can finish the following sentence and see what comes up for me? "I need pain to help me grow because..."*

(By answering this, I might find some unconscious programming I could release.)

April 21

> *"What people say is a reflection of them, not you."*
> —*PersonalDevelopmentZone.com*

To be free of the opinions of others can be a hard nut to crack. It would serve me well to understand that actually experiencing the freedom of non-attachment from anything can come and go.

Some days I'm more secure than others. I feel more content and I rattle less easily. Someone can say something insensitive, and it rolls off of me like water on a duck. Other days I feel insecure, I'm less content, and I rattle easily. Someone says something insensitive, and I need to phone a friend because I'm so hurt.

This is part of the human condition. When I remind myself of this, I'm more accepting of myself and my ups and downs. The more this happens I can even find more of my sense of humor about myself, and then I have the magical experience of when someone says something it simply rolls off. Then I know I'm free.

THOUGHT FOR THE DAY*: What if today I can practice embracing all of me?*

April 22

"Take a moment and appreciate how far you've come." —Mary Mark

---

Taking a moment to notice all of my little wins is so important, and yet often gets missed. They are there, they just rarely get airtime. If I don't make it a practice to take in my little wins, they get missed, and then I think nothing is getting better for me.

When I give attention to the little wins I have, I give them airtime. When they get airtime, over time I see the things changing for me. This continues to grow and expand for me. It impacts how I feel about myself and how I see myself. My self-esteem grows and my resting thought rate is much more positive.

I catch myself more when I circle the drain with my thoughts and interrupt them more. This allows me to slow the momentum of my negative spiraling. The more I practice this, the more positive momentum expands in my life.

This becomes a life well-lived by me. I like this idea a lot.

THOUGHT FOR THE DAY*: Giving airtime to my little wins is a huge win.*

April 23

"When you let go of being perfect, you give yourself the chance for things to happen."

—Unknown.

Perfectionism is the slow death of my spirit. It creates many ills in my life. It can make me a snarky, bitter person, or it can make me a shell of myself. Someone who cowers in the corner as my wounded inner child runs my show.

Yet when I start to reparent my wounded inner child, this has the power to change everything for me.

A great way to do this is to get a photo of myself from when I was child and place it anywhere that can help me tune into this part of me. I can make it my screensaver on my phone and computer, or hang it in my bathroom, bedroom, on my refrigerator, or just some private place that works for me, as long as it's a place where I can see and connect with this little me.

When I connect with my child self in this way, I could try to say mean things to this part of me and I bet I would find that hard, which is good. I treat myself in very harsh and unkind ways, but it's harder to see it because I'm not making the connection that it's the part of me that is wounded doing the things the bully in my brain judges me for.

Making this distinction by using a photo of my younger self is huge. If I stick with it, it becomes a lot harder to allow my inner bully to keep it up. I intervene and interrupt the bully more on my inner child's behalf.

Over time this is truly transformational for me because I am reparenting the wounded child in me and giving my inner child a new childhood. The beauty is that my subconscious doesn't know the difference. I'll notice that I'm kinder to myself and more compassionate about my supposed flaws and foibles. This is where real change can begin and with a lot more ease.

THOUGHT FOR THE DAY: *What if today I can find a photo of myself as a child and connect with this part of me?*

April 24

> *"I believe things cannot make themselves impossible." —Stephen Hawking*

Wow! This is a new perspective. How true it is that some 'thing' can't make itself impossible. Going with this, something being seen as impossible is just a well-practiced thought pattern.

This thought pattern might feel like a rock-solid truth, but what if it's still just a well-rehearsed thought pattern?

This is where tapping can come in so handy. It helps me to interrupt even the most entrenched thought patterns. The more I interrupt these thoughts, the more likely they are to lose their hold on me.

I see evidence this is happening for me as I notice these thoughts feel even a little less true. I notice one day that I'm feeling a little lighter and a little freer around some thoughts that have felt impossible to change. I might notice that circumstances in my life shift and change.

I get intuitive hits to make a phone call, or send an email, or sign up for a course, and then suddenly that well-entrenched belief (thought pattern) is no longer true for me.

THOUGHT FOR THE DAY: *What if today, when I catch myself affirming something is impossible, I can interrupt this thought pattern with tapping, even if just for a minute?*

April 25

> "When you focus on the good, the good
> gets better." —OurPositive.com

This takes practice. This isn't about saying affirmations that my brain might not believe at this stage. It's drilling down to the tiniest little nuances I can find to feel some gratitude about. Things like:

The person waved me into traffic.

The cashier smiles at me.

My cat jumped on my lap and purred.

The shoes on my feet keep my feet supported.

My pillow supports me while I sleep.

My bed feels cozy right now.

This warm tea feels good going down.

Those flowers smell good.

I loved hearing a bird sing.

These types of things. Not a long, lengthy list of all of my accomplishments; just these simple, little things. This is the way I build up my grateful muscle. It's not a race either. It's a journey that reaps incredible rewards.

If I'm having a hard time, I can look for the tiniest little thing to feel OK about (this way I don't even have to reach for what feels good), and that is a great start.

THOUGHT FOR THE DAY: *What if today, no matter how my day is, I can find one little thing to feel good or okay about? What if this is enough?*

April 26

"Perfectionism is self-abuse of the highest order." —Annie Wilson Schaef

Back to that pesky perfectionism. I cannot be reminded of this enough. Especially in a world that airbrushes and edits advertising to a crazy standard that even the models don't achieve.

If I'm judging my insides by other people's outsides, I will likely always lose. If I look at the highlight reels of others, especially on social media, and judge my life against their highlights, I'm bound to think I'm just not measuring up. Whenever I compare, I lose, and comparison is the rocket fuel beneath the wings of perfectionism.

So I think I will fire myself as the gatekeeper of being perfect.

What if I can remind myself that I'm not meant to be perfect? If I'm still on planet Earth, in a body, it's a foregone conclusion that if I drop out of the perfectionist class my culture teaches, I'll remember I'm a work in progress and will continue to be while I'm here.

I like this idea a lot better than abusing myself using comparing and perfectionism to do so.

THOUGHT FOR THE DAY: *What if today I can unhook when I notice I'm in comparing mode*

?

April 27

"Progress not perfection." — from the 12 Steps

I can use this reminder every day, throughout the day. Progress not perfect. When I come from this place, I'm far more likely to see the ways I am changing and the progress I am making. There's no place I will arrive. There's no finish line I will cross and be complete. I might finish something, but then something else will come up that I then move towards.

This is also a great reminder that if I feel stuck in a spot, and I've tapped on it, I might be being guided to hand it over to God, the Universe, Source, The Great Spirit, The Authentic Self. Whatever works for me.

As I learn to do this, I see how my life can unfold in ways so much better than I can conjure up. I find that support and help come just when I need it. Life unfolds before me with less stress and more ease.

THOUGHT FOR THE DAY*: What if today I can remember that progress is a marker far greater than perfection?*

April 28

"The Power of Yet - I don't get it…yet. I can't do this…yet. This doesn't work…yet."

—*Andrea Banks*

How brilliant is this? And what a relief. I can finish many sentences with the word yet.

I don't know…yet.

I'm not there…yet.

I haven't gotten an answer…yet.

Just adding that yet is so powerful. It suspends judgement, even if just for a moment, and it helps me to see something in a new way. It rekindles hope.

I can use The Power of Yet whenever and wherever I need to, and it feels so much better, even if just for a moment. The beauty is it's a pattern interruption. The more I use The Power of Yet, the more I find relief, and the more I find relief, the more things change for the better for me.

THOUGHT FOR THE DAY: *What if today I can use The Power of Yet, whenever and wherever I need to?*

April 29

"It's impossible…without God."
—Tosha Silver

Here's another one similar to The Power of Yet, but it's possibly even more powerful depending on my belief system. Let me try it out:

This is impossible…without God.

This will never change for me…without God.

It's hopeless…without God.

I'll never find a way without God.

"Without God" also brings me relief and is also pattern interrupting. I can change the word God to Source, Universe, The Great Spirit, The Great Self, Expanded Awareness, Fred Flintstone, the Dinosaurs, The Cabbage Patch Kids. Whatever works for me.

Just like The Power of Yet, I can use "Without God" at the end of any sentence I need to, to bring me relief, and just like The Power of Yet, the more I do this, the more things change for the better.

THOUGHT FOR THE DAY: *What if today I can use "Without God" whenever and wherever I need to?*

April 30

"All procrastination is fear."
—Elizabeth Gilbert

Glory, Hallelujah! Someone is finally expressing what procrastination is. It's so often seen as a pathology to be eradicated from my being, but procrastination is fear. On an unconscious level I am attempting to protect myself.

I might have a fear of being seen because I was publicly humiliated when I was a child and made an unconscious vow to never be seen. In this way, I am protecting my wounded child from further harm. I can take anything that I procrastinate about and find fear below the surface.

There is one other option, though, that needs to be addressed around procrastination. Sometimes I procrastinate about something because it doesn't resonate with me.

It's not that I don't want to do it, it's just that it's non-resonant and I have something else I prefer instead. As well, procrastination isn't a pathology that needs to be overcome. It's either protecting me from something my inner child fears, or my adult self just plain doesn't resonate with what's being dished up.

Either way, I'm so ready to release the belief that procrastination is something lazy people do.

THOUGHT FOR THE DAY: *What if today I can remind myself if I'm procrastinating about something, it's because I'm either trying to protect my inner child or it just doesn't resonate with me?*

May

May 1

You say I'm too sensitive like it's a bad thing. ~ Marti Murphy

---

Being too sensitive can mean I'm easily triggered when I feel criticized. If this is the case, then it's good for me to look into what the trigger is trying to show me. It's often related to a childhood event where I found myself in a hyper-critical environment and was told I was too sensitive when someone was being too insensitive with me.

So there it is. Two players in this sensitivity game. One is the offensive player wielding judgment and criticism to avoid their inner world. The other player is reactive and defensive to avoid their inner world. Both players play their part in this game of life. If either or both become conscious of their unconscious programming, then true change can happen.

The challenge is that most of us were raised to seek answers outside of ourselves. We're taught to look to others to behave differently than they do. This is always an emotional trap for any of us wanting someone to be anything other than who they are. It's a lifelong process of awakening to the programming that's running our show, but it's a journey worth taking because of the emotional freedom that can continue to develop in us.

Ironically, when one player in this game becomes conscious and shifts, eventually the other player has to shift and does so unconsciously, or they just move on.

To me, being sensitive is a wonderful quality and one that is far too out of balance in our current world. As I attend to my triggers with tapping, I free myself from the emotional congestion that's been buried in my body. As I find relief from the emotional congestion, I feel lighter and freer over time. This leads me to learning to embrace my sensitivity for the wonderful quality it is (e.g., being sensitive to the emotions of others gives me the ability to be more empathetic), without the emotional triggering.

THOUGHT FOR THE DAY: *What if my sensitivity is a much-needed blessing?*

May 2

"Feelings come and go like clouds in a windy sky. Conscious breathing is my anchor."

~ Thich Nhat Hanh

This is such a profound truth, and yet it's something that is not taught in the world. If I wasn't encouraged to feel whatever emotions I have fully in the moment, I'm experiencing them, I can find them overwhelming. It's highly likely I had all the "don't feel too much" platitudes spewed at me. How could it be otherwise in this world?

147

Like anything new, I have to learn how to allow myself my own unique emotional journey, independent of anyone else's view. This is my pathway to freedom, and to honoring myself and my experience more fully.

Tapping is a powerful way to allow myself to go into the mire of stuck emotions so I can allow my emotions to do what they are intended to do—move through me. To come and to go. This is such a practice in a world that constantly tells me to "be strong," a.k.a., don't feel so much or you'll make us all uncomfortable. It's a journey of emotional liberation well worth the trip.

THOUGHT FOR THE DAY: *What if today, if I'm feeling emotional about something, I can practice just allowing it, even if just for a minute?*

May 3

One can be the master of what one does, but never of what one feels.

~ Gustave Flaubert

Feelings come and go, if allowed. This wasn't clear to me. It's likely that I was taught to hide or suppress them. These suppressed emotions need to be attended to first, and they are likely feelings that have buried for a while.

As I use tapping to access my subconscious programming around emotions, I release them. The by-product of doing this is that I become more emotionally intelligent and thus more emotionally fit.

This process isn't about me mastering my emotions. That's a concept of the ego actually; the belief I somehow need to master my emotions. Now acceptance of all of my emotions is transformational. This allows all emotions to be acceptable and none to be forbidden.

Through this acceptance I find freedom and liberation on the other side. How wonderful can that be? My goal is not to master my emotions, but to allow and accept them. This helps my actions to become far more congruent with my emotions rather than having actions flare up that might be deemed as inappropriate (when they are actually a by-product of non-acceptance).

THOUGHT FOR THE DAY*: What if today I can practice accepting any emotion that surfaces? If I hear the bully in my brain give me push back about any emotion, I know what to tap on.*

May 4

Anyone who has a continuous smile on his face conceals a toughness that is almost frightening." ~ Greta Garbo

I've met people like this, and interestingly maybe I've met spiritual people like this. Everything is happy thoughts and being positive, to their demise.

Happy thoughts and being positive are wonderful things, but if they are used to gloss over real, genuine, heartfelt emotions that might seem negative or not of the happiest nature, then something gets missed here. This is where the frightening piece comes in. What is being witnessed is an intense suppression of emotions to stick to the positive and this is spiritual bypass. Only positive or happy thoughts are allowed, and this is like cutting off a limb or taking out an organ essential to living.

I want to learn to allow all of my emotions full expression without guilt and shame. Initially I must attend to my guilt and shame to help soften them so I can feel more fully.

The amazing thing about feeling fully is I get to know myself better. This creates more self-confidence as I learn who I really am and what's true for me. I need not pretend or be pleasing to anyone else. I get to be me, and if someone doesn't like that, I get to be good with that. This is liberation.

THOUGHT FOR THE DAY: *What if today I can ask myself, "What do I really think? What do I really feel throughout the day?" and see what comes? I need not search for an answer. I ask and just do my best to let go and see what awakens within me.*

May 5

*That was one of the saddest things
about people--their most important
thoughts and feelings often went unspoken
and barely understood. ~ Alexandra
Adornetto*

This is so true in this world I live in. We're not taught to allow feelings to be felt fully. It's more like move on from them as quickly as you can.

I might notice that some people get uncomfortable if I am expressing certain thoughts and feelings. This isn't their fault. They, like me, are a product of this culture I live in. Some people are so enculturated in not feeling they say things like:

"Just let it go."

"Get over yourself already."

"Don't take it personally."

"You think too much."

"You're too sensitive."

I might have heard these things enough I believe I'm too sensitive or I think too much, but what if that's how I'm built? I don't want to deny who I am any longer. I want to be more me than ever before. I want to discover my authentic uniqueness and be whatever that looks like more fully each and every day. If this means people leave my life because of that, I can learn to work with that. The beauty is I will call forward into my life people who love the authentic me, and that's magic in the making.

THOUGHT FOR THE DAY: *What if today I can pick one aspect of myself that I want to nourish and just give it time and attention?*

May 6

But feelings can't be ignored, no matter how unjust or ungrateful they seem.

~ Anne Frank

I might have a history of trying to ignore my feelings. It wouldn't be surprising either. It's just part of the world I live in.

This is where emotions can take on a forbidden quality, which means certain emotions are acceptable to feel while others are not. Think about anger for women and sadness for men. They are forbidden, and it's all learned.

Tapping is a great tool to assist me in going deeper into my emotions. To do so in a safe, healthy, and private way. This can be a great way to start.

This isn't a race. It's a journey I can walk throughout my life.

As I learn to allow more of the off-limit emotions in a safe and healthy way, I learn to allow all of my emotions to be expressed. I learn to allow them with reverence and with presence, and this helps me to become more emotional fit.

It's a practice, like learning anything new.

THOUGHT FOR THE DAY: *What if today, I can find a safe and private moment to allow myself an emotion that I've been telling myself I shouldn't feel?*

May 7

My feelings are too loud for words and too shy for the world. ~ Dejan Stojanovic

Feelings can come out loud when I start tapping. This is because I'm actually unearthing the emotions stored in my body and my energy system. These can come out in a big way with big emotional discharges. This is a good thing. It also helps me to understand that big, loud emotional releases are helping me to become more emotionally fit and therefore more emotionally intelligent.

I notice little changes first. Maybe I'm less reactive. Maybe I laugh off things that used to send me reeling. Maybe I'm not disturb about things that used to disturb me. Maybe I have those magical times when I say just the

153

right thing in the just the right moment because my emotional body is tuned up with regular tapping.

When I need assistance with tapping through something that's particularly large and maybe even supercharged for me, I get the support. Between that support I have this tool that's literally right at my fingertips that can help me move through life's challenges with a lot less emotional static. Tapping also allows me to speak my truth when I need to instead of stuffing my emotions. Stuffing emotions only hurts me and now I need not do it. As I allow the free expression of my emotions, I come out the other side better for it.

THOUGHT FOR THE DAY: *What if today I tap and just talk to myself about something that's been bothering me?*

May 8

To hide feelings when you are near crying is the secret of dignity. ~ Dejan Stojanovic

Dignity is beyond overrated. It is. If hiding my feelings is what it takes to have dignity, I'll pass.

If I'm talking to someone who doesn't listen and doesn't care to listen, it's pointless to keep pushing any agenda in these circumstances. However, I might have a history where I felt the only way I could be heard was to push, but maybe that still didn't get me anywhere.

When someone I'm dealing with is cut off from their emotions, or is "trying" not to feel, the only way they can maintain control is to cut me off emotionally, and if I keep trying to get them to understand me, I hurt me.

I can find a safe space to allow myself all I need to say to them in the most unedited way without them being involved. What this does for me is it allows me to be free from stuffing my emotions when I want to scream or just be heard. I get to hear me. I get to give myself my truth. I keep going into this safe space until I find relief and feel lighter.

This is a powerful way to deal with my emotions when I need to, and the other person isn't capable of that. The benefit is that I start to be less reactive and more centered, over time, around this person. This is how I set myself free. Truly I'm the only one who can give that to myself.

As it often happens, when I unhook from needing someone else to hear me, they do become available for that. It's weird how that works. Because I have given myself my truth, this gets reflected back in the outside world. I have freed myself from attachment to someone else.

THOUGHT FOR THE DAY: *What if today I can give myself my unadulterated truth about a topic that's been sticking with me for a while now? I tap and express myself fully and get support if I need it.*

May 9

Never apologize for showing your feelings. When you do, you are apologizing for the truth. ~ José N. Harris

Maybe I never thought about it like this before. When I apologize for my feelings, I am apologizing for my truth. I'm allowed my truth. I might have to take that in, but I am allowed my truth.

Learning not to apologize for my truth is another part of this. I may have a lot of practice in apologizing unnecessarily. I might have learned to do this to survive in my family of origin if I wasn't allowed to express a different viewpoint.

If I grew up in a dogmatic system where everyone was programmed to believe the same thing, I can run up against a lot of push back when I try to break free. This is where getting support can come in handy. It can help to have someone reflect back that I'm okay and I deserve my truth, even if others don't agree.

When I'm first getting used to this idea, it can be challenging because self-doubt can rule, but the more support I get, the more practice I get, and the more tapping I do, I find an inner confidence I didn't know was in me.

It's always been there actually, it just got covered over by the loudness of a world that sees things in a different way.

It takes practice, but it's doable and oh so worth it.

THOUGHT FOR THE DAY: _Today my mantra can be, "I deserve my truth."_

May 10

Just ask how I'm feeling, I want to say.
Just ask and I may tell you. But no one does.

~ Melina Marchetta

This is an all too common occurrence in a system that is fast-paced and preaches, "Get over yourself."

The world I live in can be very shaming about speaking my truth and feeling fully. If that's my experience, what if I'm being called to tune into myself about how I'm feeling. What if, as I learn to give myself my presence, I feel better and I need to be heard less and less from the outside world or from those around me.

Again the irony with me honoring me is that I have people in my experience that want to listen —that want to hear me.

When I give to myself what I'm seeking from outside of me, I usually get what I need. So funny how that works.

THOUGHT FOR THE DAY: *What if today I can take 5 minutes and practice presence with myself?*

May 11

> *When you experience loss, people say you'll move through the 5 stages of grief.... Denial, Anger, Bargaining, Depression, Acceptance..... What they don't tell you is that you'll cycle through them all every day.*
>
> *~ Ranata Suzuki*

Maybe by now, I do understand that grief is not linear. It goes back and forth between these stages for as long as I need it to. The other piece of this is grief doesn't have an expiration date. Though wallowing in grief will keep me a prisoner to it, actively allowing myself to feel it and using tapping to help me process and release it allows the journey of grief to be one that doesn't consume me. I allow it to burn through me like a fever that needs to run its course.

If anyone suggests that I should be over it, I can remember this is my journey through grief, no one else's, and we are not all cut from the same cloth emotionally.

If others become uncomfortable around my grief and want me to be over it, I can remind myself this person is not someone I should share this journey with and move on.

Grief can be a very demanding journey, but if I allow the space for it, I move through even the most demanding moments with presence and patience with myself.

THOUGHT FOR THE DAY: *My journey through grief is just that, my journey and no one else's, and I honor that today.*

May 12

Do you imagine the universe is agitated?
Go into the desert at night and look at the
stars. This practice should answer the
question. ~ Lao Tzu

Maybe I was raised to believe in a very human God. One that's the master and commander of crazy town. One minute this God loves me with deep, abiding love, but the next minute, if I misstep, the wrath of God is blown all over my being.

Is this a God I can trust and believe has my back? Maybe my image of God, or whatever I want to call it, needs a serious upgrade. Does God or the Universe have human characteristics? And if it does, why does it seem that it's the worst of the worst of human characteristics? The upgrade would be to a force that has my back. A force that guides and directs me. A force that, if I can learn to tune back into my authentic self, I feel this love and support from. A force that gives me guidance and direction through impulses to act or to move forward. What if I follow these impulses and, before I know it, my life unfolds in amazing ways? Ways far greater than my small self can imagine.

Maybe I do need to step outside under the vast expanse of stars that is above me and feel what comes. I think if I keep doing this, I might find I feel a peace and contentment independent of what the world tells me it should be like.

THOUGHT FOR THE DAY*: What if sometime today I can step outside and just pause and take in the natural world around me? Looking up into the sky is enough.*

May 13

> *When you care about someone, you can't just turn that off because you learn they betrayed you. ~ Paula Stokes,* Liars, Inc.

This is so true, and yet so challenging. If I've spent a lot of time with someone and I have a view of them or a story about them that I've been living out for a while now, if something breaks down my beliefs about someone, it's a traumatic event.

I get folded with emotions and confusion and disbelief. I've actually entered a grieving process.

I might feel enraged, then sad, then heartbroken. I might want to see them or miss them if they're not around, and then I might judge myself for this. But feelings for someone don't typically just get turned off with ease. That's the journey. To still love someone but also know that the way it's been is now over, forever.

I might establish a new normal over time that's even better, or I might not. Either way, what's important is to honor my experience and the emotions that go with that. If I catch myself judging myself, then I can tap to help myself find relief. If someone else judges me, I can do the same.

Once again, this is my unique journey—no one else's—and as I honor me, I heal.

THOUGHT FOR THE DAY: *Whatever is happening in my world today, I want to practice honoring me.*

May 14

She had power over the most
magnificent forces on Earth, but she still
didn't feel like she had power over the most
important thing of all—her own heart.

~ Josephine Angelini, Goddess

Should I have power over my own heart, or should I learn how to open my heart to myself? If I learn to make myself the most important person in my life, then I am opening my heart to myself.

161

As I learn to be more self-accepting, then I open my heart. Isn't this the love affair of a lifetime to love myself and all parts of me? Flaws, foibles, and all?

What if I can ask for guidance and direction, if I need to, as to how to open my heart to myself?

Tapping actually can clear out the learned limits I've placed on myself to survive. As I learn to release more of these limitations, I actually find I am more self-accepting, and self-acceptance eventually leads to self-love.

THOUGHT FOR THE DAY*: Trying to love myself doesn't work, but I can learn to accept all of me and then self-love just comes with ease.*

May 15

Feelings are something you have; not something you are. ~ Shannon L. Alder

---

What a great reminder. Feelings are just like thoughts; both come and go. It's when I attach to my feelings, they seem to become me because I actually haven't completed the feelings. I haven't been able to allow them to be felt and released, so they stay stuck in me, and it feels like I am my feelings.

I can hear myself saying things like:

"I'm a just a mess."

"I'm too sensitive."

"I'm an angry person."

"I'm too emotional."

When I hear statements like these, it's an indicator that I'm associating my feelings with who I am. As I allow myself to feel my emotions, and use tapping to assist me in completing emotions, they no longer rule me. Overtime, they literally become things I have rather than something I am.

THOUGHT FOR THE DAY: *Feelings move through me. I can help them do this by tapping through them and completing them.*

May 16

---

*You can't make yourself feel positive,
but you can choose how to act, and if you
choose right, it builds your confidence.* ~
Julien Smith

Making myself feel positive is spiritual bypass at its most impressive. It's often called toxic positivity. This is when I use a happy attitude that I'm not actually feeling to bypass something negative.

So I think I might not want to make myself feel positive. With tapping, I'm encouraged to go zero dark thirty. Go into the darkness of suppressed thoughts and expose them to the light. By doing this, I find I feel a lot less negative. When I feel a lot less negative, positive feelings just come. My resting thought rate is a lot more positive and uplifted without me having to "try" to be positive.

For years, tapping practitioners just tapped on the truth with people, which often came off negatively, and yet people got better. People felt better. Why would this be?

As we release the negative, we make space for who we are to come through. So our natural innate positive self comes through, much like the sun shining through once the clouds are cleared out.

THOUGHT FOR THE DAY*: I need not try to feel positive. As I honor my truth and release my truth, I find I'm naturally more positive.*

May 17

But you know Hajime, some feelings cause us pain because they remain.

~ Haruki Murakami

There is such wisdom in this statement. As Janice Berger states, "Feelings are buried dead, they're buried alive."

Unexpressed emotions get buried in the body. This isn't the place I want them to stay. If ever there's an incentive to feel more fully, this is it. My feelings don't remain if they are felt through to their completion. Learning to allow myself the fullest expression of my emotions is key.

Honoring that I probably grew up being trained to do the opposite is a step in that direction. Of all the things I may have heard about emotions, many taught me to suppress in an effort to appear strong or appear like I can control myself. Yet anyone who has felt the true depth of an emotion knows this takes absolute courage, especially when the world tells a different story.

The good news is I can learn to allow myself a fuller expression of my emotions. Tapping is a highly effective tool that helps me to do this in a deeper way.

THOUGHT FOR THE DAY: *What if today I can pick an emotion and tap for 5-10 minutes on this and see what happens?*

May 18

> *"Do not be disappointed if no one appreciates your true feelings, because they do not deserve them." ~ M.F. Moonzajer*

This can be a hard-learned lesson. The reason it can be hard is because I live in a world that actually teaches me to look to others to understand me or to appreciate me.

We want to have people in our lives who do understand and appreciate us, but the challenge is having expectations that anyone "should" understand or appreciate us. The expectations create a sense of needing it to be so.

The people in my life that don't understand or appreciate me are often my greatest teachers. They become this because they reveal my wounds. If I just keep eliminating people from my life and never seek to heal the wound, I will deal with a similar personality or circumstance again and again.

This is never because I'm doing something wrong or being punished, it's because I'm meant to see, accept, and even love the wounded part of me. This is the wounded child within me who would do anything to be loved. The part of me that will grasp and try to control someone else's behavior to feel okay.

As I learn to accept the part of me, I may judge the most, I find relief, and in this relief I find peace of mind. The gift is that I do find more people in my life who understand, accept, appreciate, and love me just as I am because I love me just the way I am.

THOUGHT FOR THE DAY*: What if today I can practice a moment of sending the part of me I judge some acceptance?*

May 19

---

*People who keep stiff upper lips find
that it's damn hard to smile.*

— Judith Guest, Ordinary People

This is such an act of suppressing emotion and never completing the emotion. Maybe I've had times where I've done this, and I've been able to feel the physical force of my suppressed emotions in my body. I literally felt this pressure building the more I tried to keep that stiff upper lip.

I might make it through the situation I find myself in, in the moment, but the time will come where I do something as simple as stick two hangers together and I go into full-blown rage. Then suddenly I'll judge myself as being crazy or unbalanced. If I behave this way in front of someone else, they might tell me how crazy they think I am too.

This is a classic example of what the by-product of keeping that stiff upper lip looks like. The emotions I feel have to go somewhere at some point. It will always seek a way to find completion, so it's better that I do so consciously rather than telling myself repeatedly that I need to control myself and my emotions only to blow up later.

With tapping, I get to let loose. I get to tap through my most potent emotions and find emotional freedom and liberation on the other side. This practice allows me to complete even the ancient emotions from early in my life.

Overtime, I will notice that my emotions feel more balanced, especially as I learn to attend to my emotions in the moment. This helps me to become more emotionally fit and intelligent.

This creates more self-confidence. This happens because I'm literally changing my physiology, and that has the power to change everything for me.

THOUGHT FOR THE DAY*: What if today I can practice tapping the moment I find I feel emotionally activated? Even if just for a minute.*

May 20

One can never ask anyone to change a feeling.

~ Susan Sontag

If there was ever an oversight in our solar system, this is it. To tell someone they shouldn't feel what they are feeling. This is the ultimate mind mess, and yet it's all too common in the world.

It's highly likely that I've been told I shouldn't feel what I'm feeling. The interesting thing is that the person that's telling me that is likely very uncomfortable with me having my emotional experience. One way to stop our discomfort is to get someone else to change. The problem is this never has lasting results. It can backfire in a red-hot minute.

What if just me reading this wakes me up to the idea that I'm 100% entitled to my feelings, no matter what they are and no matter when or how they show up?

With tapping I give this to myself in a safe and healthy way, and this allows me to give myself permission for all of my emotions.

As I learn to embrace all of my emotions, I relax and own my emotions without the self-judgement. When I do this, no emotions are off-limits especially when tapping. As I learn to honor what might even seem to be the darkest of emotions while tapping, these emotions leave my body and I do not need to act out because I'm learning to feel fully and freely.

THOUGHT FOR THE DAY: *What if any feeling I have is okay?*

May 21

"Feelings are for the soul what food is for the body."

~ Rudolf Steiner

What a concept. This is rarely taught in my culture. The truth is most of us got wired backwards about emotions. We're taught these select emotions are acceptable, while these other emotions are unacceptable.

It's never the emotion that is unacceptable. The repression of emotions is the very thing that creates actions that do harm.

When I learn to allow the emotions I feel from this amazing palette of emotions I came into this world with, I realize that my feelings are food for my soul.

I go through emotional experiences, eyes wide open and feeling fully, and then finish each emotional experience and gain so much wisdom from doing so. I get to be the fully loaded emotional being I'm meant to be as a human.

As I learn to be open to all I'm meant to experience emotionally, my soul has the space to speak to, guide, and direct me through this life experience. Then, I am never alone.

THOUGHT FOR THE DAY*: My emotions feed my soul.*

May 22

"Their feelings were suppressed so carefully in everyday life, forced into smaller and smaller spaces, until seemingly minor events took on insane and frightening significance. It was permissible to touch each other and cry during football matches."

~ Sally Rooney

This is what suppressing emotions offers. The more I suppress, the more these emotions seek an outlet. This is when I can find myself where my emotions seem to explode all over the place. I might be on the job and something seemingly innocuous happens and I find myself in an emotional downpour. This makes sense, and if seen for what it is, I can realize this is the way my emotions are seeking an outlet.

If I use tapping to address these explosions of emotions, or whatever ways my emotions are seeking an outlet, I understand that there's nothing wrong with me; my emotions just need attention.

As I give my emotions the attention and presence they deserve, I feel better. Over time, I have less and less emotional explosions. I can get to where I'm behaving in such an emotionally fit way, I may need to pinch myself to be sure this is me now. And it is. And it's a wonderful realization.

THOUGHT FOR THE DAY: *The next time I act out emotionally, what if I can remind myself this is just my emotions seeking expression? It's a great starting point.*

May 23

"Feelings are feelings. They don't have dumb or smart labels."

~ Cherise Sinclair

The only reason feelings have ever been labeled as dumb or smart, or any other such nonsense, is because I live in a culture that's not comfortable with much emotional expression. This culture would love for me to keep my shit together because that somehow means I'm more put together.

In a world that preaches this, I too have likely learned to reject, disown, or label my emotions which just adds insult to injury.

Feelings are just feelings. The more I learn to allow them and move through them, the less I need to buy into society's good or bad, right or wrong, smart or dumb labels for emotions, and the freer I will be.

THOUGHT FOR THE DAY: *Today I want to be free of labels of any kind.*

May 24

---

*"Feelings are not supposed to be logical.
Dangerous is the man who has rationalized
his emotions." ~ David Borenstein*

I might think my feelings rather than feel them. What this means is I experience a genuine emotion and I'm virtually programmed to zip up into my head and get rational about my emotions.

When I do this, I don't actually feel them. Rationalizing emotions is a great way to avoid actually experiencing them.

If, however, I learn to sit with an emotion through an experience and go into it, I will find that my emotions do what they are meant to do—move through me. They don't set up camp in my being or my body and create all manner of ills for me.

Emotions are never meant to be dangerous. They're just meant to be felt fully. If I'm someone who rationalizes my emotions, the first thing to do is to acknowledge this and attempt to send the emotional rationalizer in me some loving kindness. As I do this, I loosen the grip of my self-judgement, which allows me to feel more fully and be freed.

THOUGHT FOR THE DAY: *What if, the next time I catch myself rationalizing my emotions, I send this part of me some acceptance without changing a thing?*

May 25

"Your emotions are the slaves to your thoughts, and you are the slave to your emotions."

— *Elizabeth Gilbert*

Well, I don't want to stay a slave to my emotions, and the truth is I don't have to. The only reason I've been a slave to my emotions is because I've learned to make myself wrong for feeling many emotions the world I live in says are bad.

The remedy to this craziness is to notice my thoughts and then ask myself who I believe is running my show right now. Just asking this question does three important things:

1) It's a pattern that interrupts my thinking (which is huge).
2) It creates a space to question whether or not I want to believe these thoughts.
3) It puts my healthy adult self back into the driver's seat.

Interrupting my thoughts brings the unconscious into my conscious awareness, which is where I can shift it.

Creating a space to question whether or not I want to believe these thoughts allows me to become the observer of my thoughts and thus my emotional reaction to them rather than being a slave to them.

The noticing and then questioning of my thoughts are me activating the healthy adult part of me.

This simple little exercise has incredible power to transform my thoughts and emotions the more I practice it.

THOUGHT FOR THE DAY*: What if today I can set the intention to catch myself just once when I'm feeling bad and ask, "who's running my show?"*

May 26

"Your emotions make you human. Even the unpleasant ones have a purpose. Don't lock them away. If you ignore them, they just get louder and angrier."

~ Sabaa Tahir

Emotional suppression can lead to depression, anger, rage... the list goes on.

Why would I have these amazing emotions in me if I weren't meant to feel each of them?

What if by learning to allow all of my emotions their due process, even the unpleasant ones, I see emotions differently? I realize that some emotions are more comfortable to feel than others, but there aren't any bad, wrong, or

175

forbidden ones. All of my emotions are part of the human experience. Learning to embrace and experience them all lends to a far richer life experience rather than continuing to put limits around what emotions are acceptable to feel and what emotions are unacceptable to feel.

Sounds suspiciously like emotional freedom. I'll have more of that please.

THOUGHT FOR THE DAY*: What if today is a day I can practice allowing a fuller expression of any emotion I feel?*

May 27

"But pain's like water. It finds a way to push through any seal. There's no way to stop it. Sometimes you have to let yourself sink inside of it before you can learn how to swim to the surface."

~ Katie Kacvinsky

This holds such a valuable truth in it.

The more I learn to go deeper, to sink deeper, into my emotional landscape, the less afraid of any emotion I become. When I allow this, I behave in a way congruent with the most emotionally intelligent part of me.

It's the going down into emotions that frees them, yet the world I live in has preached the opposite. I cannot be reminded of this enough; such is the deep programming around not feeling so fully.

Here's the big secret to emotions: Feel them fully.

Tapping provides a safety net for my emotional experiences. I get to feel and find relief and feel and release.

THOUGHT FOR THE DAY: *What if today I can find moments of emotional freedom with tapping?*

May 28

"Feel, he told himself, feel, feel, feel.
Even if what you feel is pain, only let
yourself feel." ~ ~ P.D. James

I think I might be getting the point here. Feel. Feel. Feel. This is something I can learn to do. Tapping helps me to go down deeper into my emotions and feel them.

The hair on the back of my neck might stand up when I think about going down deeper into my emotional landscape. I may be recognizing a theme here, but a part of me might be terrified of actually doing this.

What if I can go to that terrified child in me and sooth them? I can let this part of me know that it will be okay. If I do this and notice a lot of resistance, that's my roadmap on what to tap on. I get to tap on how it might feel unsafe to feel so much.

I get to tap on this as long and as often as I need to until I notice I feel a little less afraid of the thought of feeling more fully, then I get to tap more.

A point will come where I notice I feel lighter and freer around going deeper into an emotion. At this point I can get some assistance if that feels more supportive. Step by step I can get there. I can build inner trust it will be okay—even highly beneficial.

THOUGHT FOR THE DAY: *Even a little step is still a step in the right direction.*

May 29

"How you react emotionally is a choice in any situation. "

~ Judith Orloff

Why doesn't this feel true for me? I could make a case this isn't true. If you step inside my body, you'll probably agree with me.

My emotions seem to take on a life of their own. I can go from zero to sixty in a millisecond, and this happens a lot. So when I hear that my emotional reactions are my choice in any situation, that can just have me feeling worse about myself.

But I can't stop my thoughts. I just can't. My thoughts fire off and then the emotional reactions follow. I can't stop my thoughts from happening in the first place, but I can interrupt them. I might have to interrupt my thoughts a bazillion times before I notice that I'm not so reactive.

If I look at it from this perspective, I find relief and I don't feel so damn bad about myself. The more I notice first, interrupt second, the less reactive I'll be. Eventually I'll find I can pause mid-reaction and begin again, and then "choice" becomes a possibility for me.

THOUGHT FOR THE DAY*: What if today I can remind myself that I can't stop my thoughts or emotional reactions, but I can interrupt them? That's a great place to start.*

May 30

"*Evelyn: There's nothing wrong with embracing one's emotions.*

Brittany: Mom, you don't just embrace your emotions, you make love to them hard-core."

~ *Gena Showalter, Catch a Mate*

I might make love to my emotions, but if so, I came by it naturally, from my growing experiences.

Any way that went down, one thing is for sure, it's likely I've adopted cultural programming around emotions that can have me feeling saturated with emotions because none have ever been completed. I have to suppress too much and too many. The beauty is I can change that right now. I can use tapping to complete emotions by going into them. As I uncover all the programming around my emotions and how and when I'm allowed to feel them, I see my emotions differently. I learn that not everything I was taught is true. Maybe even more of what I was taught isn't true for me and therefore doesn't work for me.

Now I get to decide what's best for me around my emotions and how and when I will feel them.

THOUGHT FOR THE DAY: *What if today is the beginning of me choosing how, when, and where I feel my emotions and with whom?*

May 31

"The sun always shines above the clouds."

~ Paul F. Davis

This is me actually. I came in as the sun, loaded with emotions and the ability to know what is best for me, but I grew up in a world that helped me to forget that I am the sun. The world introduced me to clouds of thinking and beliefs that moved over my sun.

But now I am waking up from this sleep walking. I'm waking up from the things I was told were true yet aren't true for me. As I wake up, I might find I get some push back from the world and the people in it who are married to a certain way of being.

I have tapping to help me move through these experiences so as not to lose myself again. The upside is that I will find people who feel just like me. People waking up right alongside me. People who support my journey.

As I release the cloudy thinking that has covered my true nature, I find the me I have always been.

THOUGHT FOR THE DAY: *I am the sun, and the clouds are my learned limits. I can release the clouds and be fully me.*

June

June 1

"What would it be like if I could accept life – accept this moment – exactly as it is?"

~ Tara Brach

Wow!! What would that be like? Living in the moment is talked about in many spiritual and mindfulness practices. Mindfulness is based on practicing being present in the moment.

In our goal-oriented world, there's a lot of focus on the future and planning for the future. In this work with tapping I am encouraged to go into the past to clear away the cobwebs. It can get confusing.

What if tapping is a practice that can help me be more in the moment. When I am tapping, I'm typically very present in the moment, even if I'm dealing with the past or a projection into the future. That might sound crazy, but I am. I can tap and see for myself if I like. Whether tapping on the past or the future, with tapping I am in the moment as far as what I'm believing and feeling right now.

Self-acceptance is a wonderful gift that tapping can bring into my life. The more I notice how often I am judging myself, the more I can tap to find relief from this.

So what if in this moment, as I read this, I can pay attention to how my shoulders feel. Are they tense? Are they tight? Would it be beneficial to relax them and let them drop down right now?

If I followed these simple instructions, I was in the moment. I may have even been accepting of how my shoulders were feeling, because I was asking myself to lower and relax my shoulders and it likely felt good. So there I was, in the moment.

I can practice little things like this throughout the day. It's simple but difficult because it's easy to allow other things to get in the way throughout my day and not stop for even a moment to be in the moment.

I can put a reminder on my phone to practice this. I can do the dishes and ask myself to be mindful while I doing them. It's likely I'll drift in and out of being in the present moment, but that's okay. That's the practice. I might find doing these simple mindfulness practices actually helps me to be more accepting of myself without trying to be. It's worth trying.

THOUGHT FOR THE DAY: *What if I can set a reminder today to take 1-3 minutes and practice mindfulness?*

June 2

"There is something wonderfully bold and liberating about saying yes to our entire imperfect and messy life."

~ Tara Brach

Oh yeah!! This speaks to acceptance. Self-acceptance. My life is many things. Perfectly imperfect. My mind might be bombarded consistently with messages about having flawless skin, the big, beautiful home, the perfect partner, the perfect body, the perfect…fill in the blank. And that's actually all crazy if I think about it, because do I know anyone that is perfect?

If I think I do it's highly likely that I'm judging my insides by someone else outsides. I'm comparing what I believe to be my lowest moments to some else's highlight reel. That never works out for me. Ever.

What if today can be a new beginning for me. What if today I can practice actually saying "yes" to my entirely perfect imperfection, sometimes messy, sometimes pulled together, and everything in between life.

It's a great practice. I can just practice saying yes to my flaws, my foibles, my fears, my tears, my wins, my peaceful moments, my harried moments, my calm moments, all of it. I need not believe it or feel it. I just have to practice it.

THOUGHT FOR THE DAY*: What if today, I can say yes to my imperfect life? Even if I don't believe in this yet. It's a practice.*

June 3

---

*"Many people are alive but don't touch
the miracle of being alive."*

~ Thích Nhất Hạnh

So true for most of us actually…not just me. My life can be an endless to-do list. I can run from one things to next. Zipping through dishes, racing through laundry, rushing to work, rushing to daycare, running to my next appointment.

Allowing myself to chill out and take in things around me probably isn't on my bucket list. My bucket list is a list of things to do. Not a state to be in.

Many people wear the hours they spent working like a badge of honor. "I worked 60 hours this week." Someone else will reply, "I worked 80."

One upping each other on how hard we've worked, how much we've accomplished.

Have I ever heard anyone competing for how much time they spent watching sunsets, birds, butterflies, flowers, clouds? Probably not.

What if being alive…really being present for more moments of my life is powerful?

What if instead of running from one task to the next, I could practice slowing down? Just simply slowing down. Slow down my driving if I drive fast. Slow down walking through a store. Especially if I'm one who can get road rage in a store, cursing at others for how slowly they're moving.

What if this practice of just slowing down helps me to tune into and touch the miracle of being alive?

THOUGHT FOR THE DAY: What if the simple practice of slowing down, even a little bit, has a huge impact on my life?

June 4

---

*"Much of spiritual life is self-acceptance,
maybe all of it."*

~ Jack Kornfield

Acceptance. Acceptance. Acceptance. Acceptance.

A word to take in.

If I'm practicing self-acceptance, then I learn to accept mistakes I've made. I learn to soften my regrets, because I realize that anytime in my life, it appeared I made mistakes, I was doing the best I could considering where I was at mentally, emotionally, and even spiritually.

I learn to make it all okay. From this comes self-forgiveness and then…dare I say it…eventually self-love. I realize that I'm always doing the best I can in any moment. I really am. As I work with this, I realize that everyone around me is doing the best they can too, even if their best sucks for me.

I get to use tapping to help me move through the hurts I might have towards someone else's best that may not appear like their best. If I do this with consistency, I realize that they, like me, are doing the best they can, given where they are at in the moment.

I can come to this belief because I've allowed myself all of my feelings about myself and my behavior and about them and their behavior.

THOUGHT FOR THE DAY: What if self-acceptance is a practice that's made easier with tapping through my feelings about myself and others?

June 5

> *"You are the sky. Everything else is just the weather."*
>
> *~ Pema Chödrön*

Another great reminder I am so much more than I witness of myself, in this 3D world I'm living in right now. I might have heard the saying that I'm a spiritual being having a human experience and I might even believe this intellectually, but emotionally is another story.

I'm so much more aware of living in this 3D world than I am of the authentic self I truly am. Maybe I've done a lot of spiritual practices to help me remember and get tuned back into the truth of my being, but this 3D world is so real despite what all the sages, saints, and gurus have to say. It's much harder to tune into my authentic self.

A great practice to help me with this is to get out in nature more. And once I'm in nature to take it in. To sit with it and notice how amazing it is. To see the never-ending abundance of the blades of grass, to the leaves on the trees, or the grains of sand at the beach.

I've learned to be so busy with the business of life that it's easy to lose sight of what a miracle nature is. What a miracle I am. What I miracle my body is.

When I practice mindfulness in nature, I'm learning to take in the expansiveness that surrounds me every day. I pause to tune in. I might stop and listen to a bird singing its song. I might close my eyes and feel the breeze gently caressing my face. I might see the stars at night and notice how vast it all is.

The more I do this, the more I tune in. The more I tune in, the more I find feelings surfacing with a knowingness to them. Moments of hope. Moments of feeling how amazing I am and how amazing everything around me is. As I practice this, I remember that I am the sky, and all the other human stuff is just the weather.

THOUGHT FOR THE DAY*: What if today I can pause, even for a minute and take in what I miracle I am in every way?*

June 6

---

*"Mindfulness isn't difficult, we just
need to remember to do it."*

~ Sharon Salzberg

Making anything a habit, takes time. I can set reminders or put post-it notes around to help me remember to tap, to be mindful or both.

Tapping works when I do it. Mindfulness works when I practice it. I need not sit and tap for hours on end. If I just use tapping to assist in interrupting patterns of thinking causing me stress, even if just for a minute or two throughout the day, this has a cumulative effect. It's the same with mindfulness.

When I see the benefits of these practices, it can be inspiring to continue. If I don't tap or practice mindfulness regularly, it's important not to judge myself for this. This never serves me.

It's interesting that if I really let myself off the hook, the inspiration seems to come to do things that are beneficial to me.

I could be in resistance, out of an unconscious fear that's holding me back, because it's attempting to protect me. If so, then maybe I can get some help to attend to my resistance and see what happens.

Another option could be this…What if the reason I'm not doing things beneficial to me, is so I can learn to practice self-acceptance.

Since I can't change what I judge, this could make sense. Maybe it's reflecting a need to be a little kinder to myself. Maybe this is something I need to learn because it wasn't taught.

What if my truth around this will come as I ponder whether I really am in resistance to protect myself or I'm not moving because I'm being guided and directed to send myself some acceptance? Something that's been missing from my life. Either way, there's helpful information here if I learn to see it this way.

THOUGHT FOR THE DAY*: What if I can ask my authentic self to assist me in awakening to what I need to understand?*

June 7

"Mindfulness is very simple. It means you become intentionally aware of the present moment while paying close attention to your feelings, thoughts, and sensations of the body."

~ S.J. Scott

"The body never lies."

"The body is the subconscious mind."

"Your brain is not in charge.:

World-class neuroscientist, Dr. Candace Pert says your brain is not in charge. She challenges conventional science, and anyone interested in total wellness, to reconsider how our bodies think, feel, and heal.

Going with her wisdom, then mindfulness can help me to tune into the present moment and witness my feelings, my thoughts and what's happening in my body.

Tapping is another powerful tool to help me become more mindful.

As I practice both tapping and mindfulness, I live more in my body, rather than in my head.

I realize how amazing my body is. It's my constant companion through this lifetime and it carries for me all the unexpressed emotions I haven't completed.

As I learn to be mindful and tap when I need to, I integrate my body/mind/feeling connection. This allows me to live more grounded in my life. This helps me to respond more often than react because I'm soothing my nervous system.

Life becomes a lot easier. That's a big upside.

THOUGHT FOR THE DAY: *What if today, I can take 2-3 minutes and set an alarm and practice tapping, and then practice mindfulness?*

June 8

"The best way to capture moments is to pay attention. This is how we cultivate mindfulness."

~ Jon Kabat-Zinn

What if capturing a sunset fills me with good feelings? What if pausing and listen to the birds sing fills me with peace? What if I pay attention to a cup of tea I'm nursing slows me down? What if petting my cat or dog soothes me?

What if staying present with a friend I'm talking to builds genuine intimacy? What if focusing on each dish as I wash them, turns a mundane act into a peaceful experience?

What if being present with my child builds genuine intimacy? What if feeling the breeze on my face soothes me? What if feeling the warmth of my clothing on my body fills me gratitude? What if savoring each bite when I eat, slows me down and helps my digestion? I can pick anything, and practice mindfulness and see what happens. It might slow me down and help me start to take in my life instead of rushing through it.

THOUGHT FOR THE DAY: *What if I can take 2-3 minutes today and practice being mindful?*

June 9

"Don't believe everything you think.
Thoughts are just that – thoughts."

~ Allan Lokos

This is where understanding who is running my show in any given moment can become so helpful.

If I'm in a highly emotional state and feeling out of sorts, I can ask myself, 'who is running my show right now.' The potency of emotions indicates that my wounded child is runny my show. Just the noticing is a great pattern interrupt. I don't even need to tap, but I certainly can. Whatever I'm called forward to do.

If I notice that I'm feeling bad about myself because I've been "should-ing" on myself, and I ask myself 'who is running my show right now.' The punitive, judging inner dialogue indicates that the bully in my brain is in charge.

Just asking myself this, is a way to become mindful and present in the moment. Now that I've put my healthy adult self back in charge, I can decide if want to listen to the bully who's always feeding me worst case scenario, or if I want young, vulnerable version of myself to be in charge.

I now get to choose what thoughts I want to believe and what thoughts I seek to let go of.

A simple, yet powerful way to detach from my crazy inner dialogue and find peace.

THOUGHT FOR THE DAY: *What if today, I can use 'who is running my show' when needed to unhook from the firestorm of thoughts in my head that just take over?*

June 10

"When we get too caught up in the busyness of the world, we lose connection with one another – and ourselves."

~ Jack Kornfield

Truth! I can see this when I'm mindfully observe two strangers sitting together and yet both are on their phones and disconnected from each other.

I can see this in myself if I'm catch up in the 'just one more thing' paradigm that keeps me on a never-ending hamster wheel.

Just one more thing and then I'll rest.

Just one more thing and then I'll sit down.

Just one more thing and then I'll pay attention to my child.

Just one more thing and then I'll sit and enjoy my meal.

Just one more thing. Just one more thing. Just one more thing.

This is nothing less than pure madness.

THOUGHT FOR THE DAY: *What if today I can set a reminder to see when I'm in the 'just one more thing' madness and just pause and take a simple breath before I continue?*

June 11

"We cannot force the development of mindfulness."

~ Allen Lokos

Wait! What? Hang on a minute. I think I've spent a lifetime trying to force my development.

I mean think of all the pithy sayings that tell me I should...

> *"Some people want it to happen, some wish it would happen, others make it happen." ~ Michael Jordan*

This is Michael Jordan we're talking about here. I mean if I don't make it happen who will? He made everything happen.

And yet when he was on the court, I think it's safe to say, he was in the zone, in the flow. In those moments he seemed to allow something greater than his human self to move through him. These were moments of magic.

Here's another one:

> *"Infuse your life with action. Don't wait for it*
> *to happen. Make it happen. Make your own future.*
> *Make your own hope." ~ Bradley Whitford*

This sounds exhausting if I'm honest. And maybe I've tried this often and nothing comes of this action for me.

What if instead of infusing my life with action, I consider stepping back and allow the next step to come? This would be me allowing that flow that Michael Jordan always seemed to tune into, whether he was aware of it or not. (I think he was.) What about this idea? Then I'm acting from inspiration.

If I'm always pushing the agenda of my ego, I can miss the amazing flow of inspiration that's always there for me, if I just take a breath and a step back from all the pushing energy the world teaches. This sounds nicer and yet might be hard to believe. What if I can practice pausing anyway?

THOUGHT FOR THE DAY*: What if there is a better way? It might not be the familiar way, but that's okay.*

June 12

> *"Nothing ever goes away until it has*
> *taught us what we need to know."*
>
> *~ Pema Chödrön*

Damnit!! Come on now! Grrr!!!

This does seem true. I can run away from any situation, but it will return again and again in a different form with the same lesson.

This isn't to punishing me or because I'm doing something wrong.

It's just that I lost touch with my authentic self a long time ago and what if this is the way the authentic self is actually helping me to come back to this part of me.

When I shift within myself, there's incredible freedom in this.

I'm not as easily activated by things as I used to be. This is true freedom.

When I find a circumstance or behavior repeating itself, it's really for my awakening.

It's likely I got misguided and may have learned to make myself wrong when this happens because…

"I must have attracted this."

"I must not be aligned with my desires."

"I must not be a vibrational match for it."

"I must need to visual what I want happening more."

What if I've tried this to no avail? I can keep using this concepts to make myself wrong and beat myself up again, or I can decide that things keep repeating themselves because I'm still in the awakening process and this will move on, as I learn to accept and love myself and awakening to a new way.

THOUGHT FOR THE DAY: *Real change begins with acceptance for what is, exactly as it is right now.*

June 13

---

*"Mindfulness is a way of befriending
ourselves and our experience."*

~ Jon Kabat-Zinn

This sounds nice. Being mindful is a way to befriending myself. It does make sense if I think about it.

If I'm present with someone I'm interacting with, I'm being mindful and giving them the gift of my full attention.

If I'm being mindful with my own activities, I'm being present for myself. It is a gift I give to myself.

It's not something I learned, but it's something I can practice and get better at.

It's not like I have to force myself to be present all day. That would not work for me and it's putting a lot of pressure on myself, which I don't need more of.

Just taking a few minutes to practice each day is a gift I can give to myself. Over time, when I'm experiencing the benefit of this, I'll likely desire to gift myself more of this. It's soothing to my nervous system, which is always a good thing.

THOUGHT FOR THE DAY*: What if today is another day I can take 2-3 minutes and sit outside in nature and practice mindfulness? Even if this means sitting inside and looking out at nature.*

June 14

"Looking at beauty in the world, is the first step of purifying the mind."

~ Amit Ray

Oh yes. This is a perfect follow-up to yesterday. To spend more time in nature. To take in the beauty of the natural world I live in. Even if I live in a big city, I can find a park, a public garden, a tree, some flowers or even birds hanging out on buildings.

The natural world is so healing. When I take even a few minutes a day and close my eyes and feel the breeze, or watch the sunrise, I am stepping back from the world I live in everyday, all day long, that has me so busy I miss all the beauty that's around me.

My soul speaks through the natural world. I can find peace, even if just for a moment looking at a flower. Watching ducks swim around a pond. Anything like this usually has the power to soften me.

This is good for me and good for my soul.

THOUGHT FOR THE DAY: *What if today, I can spend 2-3 minutes tuning into the natural world in whatever way I can?*

June 15

"Step outside for a while – calm your mind. It is better to hug a tree than to bang your head against a wall continually." ~
Rasheed Ogunlaru

Outside again. And there's a reason for this. What would this be like to go outside and hug a tree when I'm frustrated, or sad, or lonely? What if something this simple has the power to change my state of mind in the moment? If nothing else I might get a good laugh out of it and that's definitely a state changer.

This gives a whole new meaning to being a tree hugger. Oh I think tree huggers might just know what's going on.

Stephen Colbert, the nighttime talk show host talked about, "loving the bomb." Basically what he meant was, he would be on an elevator and do something outrageous that would be embarrassing, so he could practice learning to be okay with embarrassment. The more he did this, the better able he was to do stand up and bomb on a joke and then have a great comeback that super-ceded the bomb. The joke about the bomb became the highlight. He was making light of the bomb and poking fun at his seeming 'fail' and yet his reprisal was for his comeback to have the audience roaring.

This was his salvation. What if hugging a tree can be mine? What if it's a way to lighten my emotional load and learn to take myself a lot less seriously?

I might even make someone else's day if they're witness to it and they in turn take themselves less seriously in that moment. Who knows? One thing is for sure. It's an interesting pattern interrupt.

THOUGHT FOR THE DAY: *What if today, I dare to hug a tree?*

June 16

> *"Things don't have to be perfect in order for them to be good."*
>
> *~ WholeHeartedWoman.org*

In this flawless skin, perfection seeking world, what if I can be one who is good enough. Good is great for me.

What if this changes so much more me? What I can look in the mirror and say...good enough? What if I can step on the scale and say...good enough? What if I can make my bed and say...good enough? What if I can NOT make my bed and say...good enough? What if I can make a meal and say...good enough?

203

What if I can finish many sentences with good enough and what if good enough becomes great for me?

THOUGHT FOR THE DAY*: What if whatever I do today can be good enough?*

June 17

"That's life: starting over, one breath at a time."

~ Sharon Salzberg

The do-over. This is essential what Sharon is speaking to.

If I argue with someone and I don't feel good about how I handled it, instead of allowing the bully to occupy space in my head and pound away at how I should have done it differently, I can call for a do-over. I can go to the other party and tell them I want to do a do-over. I want to go back and redo what happened but from a healthy place.

I do this for me. So I can practice doing things in a healthier way. The bonus is, if they're willing, I can effectively dissolve or at least dilute hurt feelings by own my part and then doing it in a way I feel good about.

The brain doesn't know the difference. The brain just anchors in the new behavior. The other person gets to do the same. It's helpful it both parties are willing, but if they're not, I can tell them I'm available for a do-over when them find themselves in a place to do it.

If they don't, then I can do it with myself and rewrite what happened and rewire a new habit.

THOUGHT FOR THE DAY: *I can always call for a do-over and begin again.*

June 18

"Absorb what is useful, discard what is not, add what is uniquely your own."
~HappyLives360.com

Great words and an even better idea to practice. No matter what the mass majority might say, I can find my own way. I can separate myself from the masses and find what is resonate with me and what works for me.

We're not cookie cutter humans. What works for someone else may not work for me.

What works for me may not work for someone else.

If try to fit myself into a system or a practice that doesn't resonate with me, then I dishonor me when I do this. I want to honor my own unique journey.

If tapping doesn't work for me, I can be guided to something else that does. I can ask for guidance and direction and to be shown what will work for me and then see what comes. In this way, I awaken to my not having to figure it all out right now. I can ask for guidance and ask to be shown what is for the highest good for all concerned. As I make this a practice, I might find that my life unfolds in amazing ways. I might not need a list of goals, because each step I need to take is revealed to me and I take that next step. It takes practice to learn to trust I can do this, and that life will unfold in a way that's even better than I could visualize or imagine. At least in this way, I create the space for an expanded awareness to be revealed.

THOUGHT FOR THE DAY: *What if today, if I feel confused or stuck, I can ask for guidance and direction and to be free of needing to know right now and then see what shows up?*

June 19

"A few simple tips for life: feet on the ground, head to the skies, heart open…quiet mind."

~ Rasheed Ogunlaru

This sounds amazing and yet I don't think I'm very good at this. And what if that's 100% okay.

I might be in my head a lot and not very grounded in my body, but if I allow my head to look to the sky, even if just for a moment today, I might find I feel peace. I might see a bird flying or I might see the stars sparkling away. Peace can come from such moments.

I might find I have my feet more firmly on the ground, so to speak, as I learn to listen to the inner wisdom that can come through me in quiet moments. In these moments I realize I'm not alone there is guidance available as I learn to ask for it and to allow it to come without a particular agenda as to how it should look or show up.

I might have tucked my heart away from many past hurts and yet what if I can considering opening my heart to myself. A powerful way to do this is to find a photo of myself as a child and start to look at my child self and see what I might want to say to this part of me who went through a lot. I think I might find kind words to say. This is a beginning for me to open my heart to myself. It's often easier to do it with a younger version of myself.

I might find that my mind quiets naturally as I give myself more quiet moments, like taking in the stars or watching an animal do its thing.

Simple ways to practice what Rasheed Ogunlaru is talking about.

THOUGHT FOR THE DAY: *What if I can find a photo of myself as a child and put it somewhere prominent, so I can open my heart to myself?*

June 20

"You only lose what you cling to."

~ Buddha

Clinging, gripping, grasping…all ways I have learned to try to will a certain outcome. Of course I cling…this world often pushing the ego's agenda. It's ALL up to me, of course I cling.

If, however, I can turn to God, the Universe, The Great Spirit, my authentic self, expanded awareness, then I might realize that I need not cling so hard, if I learn to loosen my gripping and turn something I've clung to over to whatever I believe in, maybe the first step is to give my version of God an upgrade from what I was taught. I'm not about to turn something over to an entity I don't trust. I might have to decide what I could trust and start there.

This is its own journey.

I may have heard…Let Go, Let God, but no one ever told me how to let go.

In a world that constantly tells me I have to make it happen, it's not surprisingly, I cling so hard.

And what if I can ask myself the following and see what comes…

"If I could release my clinging and turn this thing over, what might that feel like? If my answer tells me it doesn't feel safe, then I can tap on it not feeling safe. If my answer tells me it feels like a relief, I can tap into this feeling of relief and anchor it in a bit. Whatever resistance comes up around this, I have tapped to help me soften it. This will allow whatever messages or guidance to come to me. Over time I'll notice that I'm clinging less and trusting more because trust is being nurtured.

THOUGHT FOR THE DAY: *What if today, I can take a moment and ask myself if I trust that the Universe has my back? If not, no problem, I know what to tap on.*

June 21

> *"Nothing can harm you as much as your own thoughts unguarded."*
>
> *~ Buddha*

I may have noticed that my thoughts can tell me a crazy story of worst-case scenario often. This is when I notice my thoughts are unguarded.

The more I catch myself thinking worst case type thoughts, the more I can interrupt these thoughts and put my healthy self back in the driver's seat. I may not believe I have a healthy self in me, but I do. It's just covered over with all the worst case thinking I've adopted. As I become more conscious of my thoughts, I soften the grip they've had on me.

As my unconscious thinking becomes conscious, this is where I can attend to it and shift my thinking.

It's not actually hard, if I realize that I just have to interrupt my thinking. I need not change it. I need not try to think positive. The interrupting is enough. I can see evidence sooner than I might believe.

I also need not sit around all day paying attention to my thoughts. In the moments I do become conscious that is enough.

THOUGHT FOR THE DAY: *What if today, I can take a minute or two right now and notice what I'm thinking and interrupt if I need to?*

June 22

"Every experience, no matter how bad it seems, holds within it a blessing of some kind. The goal is to find it."

~ Buddha

If I can believe this, things can change for me.

I might have learned to lament about anything bad that happened. This is good to do if I shift the energy while I'm lamenting. Like using tapping or mindfulness.

The more I practice going into the bad and using whatever works best for me to attend to my lamenting the more I will find that a bad experience feels lighter and I feel better.

It's not something I have to attend to 24/7. Just intending to do so, can help me become more aware. This too in enough.

I will notice that I see more goodness and blessing in many bad experiences I've had without having to try to see the good. The good just starts to be revealed as the muck clears out of my psyche.

THOUGHT FOR THE DAY: *Keeping it simple is super powerful.*

June 23

"The feeling that any task is a nuisance will soon disappear if it is done in mindfulness."

~ Thích Nhất Hạnh

This is actually true if I try this. I can try this with one dish I'm washing, or washing my hands, tying my shoe, sweeping the floor, making my bed.

If I try this while taking a sip of coffee or tea, or savoring one bite, I might see it easier to begin with, but once I become mindful of this moment and what I'm doing in it, my attention does shift. I often relax and just take something in, in a deeper way.

I might notice when I'm washing the dish how nice the warm water feels on my hands or how the dish feels in my hand. I slow the racing of my mind down from the to-do list I have. I just take in this moment. That is all.

The nuisance comes from how I'm seeing it and if I'm present, I'm in the moment, not thinking about the past or what I need to do in the future. I'm bathing in this moment right here and now and I feel peace.

THOUGHT FOR THE DAY*: What if today, I can do one thing with mindfulness?*

June 24

"Do not dwell in the past, do not dream of the future, concentrate the mind on the present moment."

~ Buddha

Oh please. Really?

I live in the past and the future and why wouldn't I'm told to set goals, to create a plan of action. To just do it.

What if I can take a moment and ponder this thought from a sweet little movie, "My Life in Ruins.

212

Nia Vardalos' character Georgia asks Georgoulis character Poupi… "Don't you have goals or a plan for your life?"

He looks at her sincerely and asks her…

"How can you plan life?"

That might throw a wrench in the goal setting, action-oriented, high octane idea's that come from the world I live in.

This doesn't mean that I will be able to live my life in the moment very often, but it slows me down and opens me up to greater possibility, if I'm mindful of more moments in my life.

I might find I don't want to set goals. I might find that I'm more inclined to allow inspiration to come and then to act from this inspired place. I might find I'm living an interesting life this way and a life with less stress and more wonderful moments.

THOUGHT FOR THE DAY*: What if today I can put any goal chasing off for the day and see what happens? As I catch myself feeling uncomfortable or feeling like I need to do something about my goals I can remind myself that just for today, I'm setting this aside.*

June 25

"Just as a snake sheds its skin, we must shed our past over and over again."

~ Buddha

Releasing the past. Letting the past go. Moving beyond my past.

Tapping gives me a way to do this, yet I go into the past and attend to the emotional charges still in my nervous system and related to my past to release, let go and move beyond.

It might sound counter intuitive and it might go against spiritual practices that tell me to look towards the light, but I'm both having a human experience and a spiritual experience simultaneously and ignoring either experience puts me out of balance.

As I go into the layers of skin from my past and tap through them, I do shed them. I might have the memory still there, but the emotional charge that's been attached to this memories is released, and I feel better, lighter, and freer. I shed the skin of my past experiences and my gift is emotional freedom and who knows what else.

THOUGHT FOR THE DAY*: It's okay to revisit my past to shed a new layer of it so I can find more emotional freedom.*

June 26

> *"Peace comes from within. Do not seek it without."*
>
> *~ Buddha*

This can be a tough nut to crack. I might know this is true intellectually, but I'm programmed to believe that if people outside of me would just behave differently, I will be okay.

I might find a bazillion people who agree with me, but this still doesn't bring me peace.

In fact, I feel trapped if I buy into the belief that someone else needs to be any different than they are.

I can tap on all of my feelings around them and find relief and I can also ask for help from a power greater than my small self to help release me from any prison of needing anything outside of me to be different for me to be okay.

I need not go this alone. I do my part and tap to find release and then ask for guidance and allow inspiration to come.

I will find I have more moments where I am free of this need and my feathers are less ruffled by someone else's behavior. This is a big win for me.

THOUGHT FOR THE DAY: *What if today I can ask for guidance on how to detach from anyone or anything I'm attached to and then sit back and see what comes?*

June 27

"The art of peaceful living comes down to living compassionately & wisely."

~ Allan Lokos

Compassion for myself would be the perfect place to start. I can think of this as me being compassionate with someone I may not be ready to yet, or I can consider that the person in my life who needs the most compassion is me.

Ironically, as I practice self-compassion, I become kinder to myself. As I become kinder to myself this spills out on to other people in my life.

I'm giving to myself what I need most. This fills up my cup which then allows me to give genuine and heartfelt compassion to someone else when I'm sincerely ready to.

I need not try to be compassionate with anyone else. That never works. As I learn to be self-compassionate, I wake up to my authentic self and self-compassion leads to self-acceptance, which leads to self-love.

This is a wonderful path to my own inner awakening and its ultimate benefits others.

THOUGHT FOR THE DAY: *What if today, I can find one thing to practice self-compassion on?*

June 28

"It is never too late to turn on the light."

~ Sharon Salzberg

What a message of hope. It's never too late. I may have heard stories of people on their death bed, with a profound realization that allows them to leave in peace and feel fulfilled.

What if it's never too late for me to turn to my inner light? What if it my light is actually always on, but it just gets overlayed with the loudness of the world? What if getting quiet internally can help me tune back into my inner light? Tapping and mindfulness help me to diminish my internal noise and create the space for my inner light to shine through.

I love the idea this idea.

THOUGHT FOR THE DAY: *What if today I can tap or practice mindfulness or both to diminish my inner noise so my inner light can shine through?*

June 29

"You can't stop the waves, but you can learn to surf."

~ Jon Kabat-Zinn

Oh yes. Learning to surf the waves of my emotions. They do come in a wavelike pattern if I pay attention.

As I learn to surf the waves, I release perfectionism.

I realize that a little change is enough. A lot of little changes add up to big changes.

I learn to let life unfold rather than trying to make things happen. I learn to act from inspiration, not from the pushing place my ego comes from.

I learn to recognize when I'm in the pushing mode and step back. I learn to allow what needs to unfold to unfold.

I learn to let what needs to move on, move on.

I see the waves of life coming my way and I learn how to surf these waves in a fuller and freer way.

I release the need to control my environment and I open up to moving with what is showing up.

This happens with little daily steps. Even one moment of mindfulness a day is very helpful. Tapping when I'm experiencing an emotional charge is another step I can take. I realize there is no finish line to cross, there's just life unfolding before me and I learn to either stay in resistance to what is happening, or I can learn to use these tools to help me surf the waves of living.

THOUGHT FOR THE DAY: *What if today I can do one thing that helps me surf through what life is bringing to me?*

June 30

"Attachment leads to suffering."

~ Buddha

When I'm attached to a particular outcome and that outcome doesn't happen, it's likely that I suffer disappointment, anger, frustration, or whatever emotion shows up for me.

There's a great line from Melody Beatty, "The time to detach the most is the time you think you can't the most." Hello!!! If it were easy I would do it more often.

Learning to unhook from the idea that I'm in charge and I need to make things happen can be very challenging because it can work for a while to make it all happen.

But how do I feel when I seem to stay stuck in a cycle of trying and failing.

Am I really failing? The world would tell me I am, but am I really failing? Is it possible that whatever I think needs to happen isn't for my highest good? What if as I release the attachment to a particular outcome, I feel lighter and from this lighter feeling I find newly inspired ideas come a lot easier? What if this is the way I'm actually meant to live?

I see that when things don't appear to go the way I think they should, it's not because I'm doing anything bad, or wrong, it's because there's something so much better that needs the space to unfold.

As I learn to let go, I learn to let in the highest and best for me. This sure feels a lot better.

THOUGHT FOR THE DAY: *What if today if I notice something isn't going my way, I can remind myself that it's not working out because there's something better coming?*

July

July 1

*"You can't pour from an empty cup.
Take care of yourself first."* ~ *Unknown*

Self-care and putting myself first is becoming something that's seen as more important and yet there are still many messages in the world that teach me to put everyone in front of myself.

I'm supposed to do all, be all, see all and do it all with a smile. Sounds exhausting.

What if I can weigh in on how important it is to fill my cup up first and foremost.

"According to Living Self Care, self-care tends to improve our immunity, increase positive thinking, and make us less susceptible to stress, depression, anxiety and other emotional health issues. Taking time out to care for ourselves helps remind us and others that our needs are important, too."

I'll have more of this please. Self-care takes practice, especially if I haven't done it. The key is to take consistent baby steps. Starting small helps me to build momentum and not feel overwhelmed.

If I chose what feels good to me and just start with 2-3 minutes and then add on a minute as I feel inspired to, over time, I will build a self-care practice that's beneficially to my well-being.

THOUGHT FOR THE DAY: *What is one simple thing I can do today to be good to myself for only 2-3 minutes?*

July 2

---

*"Drink your tea slowly and reverently,
as if it is the axis on which the world earth
revolves – slowly, evenly, without rushing
toward the future; live the actual moment.
Only this moment is life."*

~ *Thich Nhat Hanh*

Oh this could be epic self-care. To sit and savory a cup of tea. It might sound easy, but if I haven't been practicing self-care, I could feel like I might crawl out of my skin even attempting this.

This awareness is part of practicing self-care. To be mindful of what's happening for me around this. Another layer of self-care.

What if I sit to savor that cup of tea, coffee, or whatever my choice is, and I notice quickly that I feel uncomfortable with this. Noticing my discomfort is practicing self-care because I'm giving myself the gift of mindfulness.

That's a win in my self-care practice and it's enough. Just the noticing, being present to my inner world.

It's not about how many hours of yoga, meditation, eating plan, etc. It's about my attention to my inner world. That's a great start and what if learning to give myself credit for this is self-care. I like it.

THOUGHT FOR THE DAY: *What if just noticing how I feel about a potential self-care practice, is actually the beginning of self-care?*

July 3

"We might begin by scanning our body.
… and then asking, "What is happening?"
We might also ask, "What wants my
attention right now?" or "What is asking for
acceptance?"

~ Tara Brach

Self-care at its finest.

I don't want my self-care practice to become yet another list of to-do's that I feel overwhelmed by. That isn't self-care. I want this to be easy for me.

If I take even a minute and do a body scan and ask myself…

What is happening in my body right now?

What needs my attention right now?

What is asking for my acceptance right now?

I am caring for myself and this is enough.

THOUGHT FOR THE DAY: *Short and simple is a great way to practice self-care.*

July 4

Every time we become aware of a thought, as opposed to being lost in a thought, we experience that opening of the mind.

~ Joseph Goldstein

This is such a simple and yet powerful way to care for myself. To notice my thoughts.

I can use this reminder all the time because it's easy to get lost in thoughts and remain unconscious to what's happening for me.

I circle the drain with my thoughts and before I know it I've got a lot of anticipatory stress building up over something that hasn't even happened yet, or something that has happened, but I can't change it.

If, however, I notice my thoughts more, I see how my thoughts are like a constant waterfall.

Even having mindful moments is huge. I need not try harder or do it better, I just have to keep being reminded that my thoughts can run amuck and I'm the one who pays the price for this.

Tapping is another tool I can use to tap through my racing thoughts because I'm very conscious of my thinking and then more can surface and be released.

This can bring me a lot more peace.

THOUGHT FOR THE DAY: *What if today, just by reading this, I might have a moment when I become conscious of what my thoughts are? What if this is enough?*

July 5

"The greatest communication is usually how we are rather than what we say."

~ Joseph Goldstein

I've been around people whose words don't seem to match their behavior.

They might say one thing, but their body language tells me something different.

It's likely that I've done this.

I want to become more congruent so what I say, matches what I do and how I act.

This takes practice, because there's a lot of programming in the world that tells me to do or be something I might not be congruent with.

When I learn to understand what I think, and what I feel, I awaken to who I am.

As I awaken to who I am, I learn how to live more congruently with my truth.

I find I feel more peace when I honor my truth regardless of what the world tells me. Getting in touch with my truth is its own journey. As I learn to unhook from what the world tells me, my authentic self has the space to be witnessed by me. It's journey worth taking.

THOUGHT FOR THE DAY*: I'd rather be my authentic self than someone else's idea of who I should be.*

July 6

> *"Emotion arises at the place where mind & body meet. It is the body's reaction to mind."*
>
> *~ Eckhart Tolle*

The body and mind are intimately connected. Disease has been linked time and time again to stress and environmental causes. When my emotions are running me my body is in a state of chronic stress. My body can experience elevated cortisol levels when I'm stressed which just raised the bar on my stress.

My body and mind are dancing together in a way where my emotions take over. Once this happens my body and emotions are pinging off of each other.

Tapping helps me to interrupt this pinging. It's changes the programming in my mind and emotions and the result is that my body calms down as my emotions calm down and my thoughts stop racing.

There is absolutely nothing wrong with me when I'm in a highly emotional state. I might have heard things like I'm a mess, or a I'm crazy, but whatever I'm experiencing is 100% normal given where I'm at in any time.

As I learn to alter my pattern of epic self-judgment, I act towards myself in kinder ways. I realize that I deserve to treat myself kindly and I learn how to.

This all can result from learning to soothe myself when I'm in an emotional upset.

This helps me to self-regulate the more I practice this. Over time, I find I'm less emotional reactive and more thoughtfully responsive.

THOUGHT FOR THE DAY*: What if today I can take 2-3 minutes and be mindful of how my emotions impact my body? How does my body respond to my emotions? It's a great beginning.*

July 7

"We are born wise. We are born complete." ~ Yogi Bhajan

What a great mantra to say to myself often. Even if I don't believe it yet.

Even if I hear a host of 'yeah but's' that's okay. The 'yeah but's' let me know what I need to tap on. What my truth is right now. My truth can be changed the more I tap through it. It might sound something like this...

I was born wise. Then why do I feel so stupid?

I was born complete. Then why do I feel so broken?

I hear what my truth is... I feel stupid. I feel broken.

This is why affirmations can actually create more of a problem for me. If I'm not mindful of the 'yeah but's' that follow them...I feel stupid...I feel broken, then I can use affirmations all day long and twice on Sunday and I find I actually feel worse. This is because whatever imprint is in place in my psyche is like a cloud that's blocking me from seeing the sun and feeling its warmth.

With this knowledge I can use affirmations to help me see where I'm at in my beliefs about myself and then tap to help shift these beliefs.

Another helpful thing I can do is add this...

What if I can learn to believe I was born wise? What if I can learn to believe I was born complete?

As I tap to soften what doesn't feel true for me and then add "What if" to an affirmation, I will find that affirmations actually feel true for me. Woo-hoo!!!

THOUGHT FOR THE DAY: *What if today I can say one affirmation and just notice the 'yeah but' that follows? I can then tap and/or change and affirmation with What if?*

July 8

"If you are willing to look at another person's behavior toward you as a reflection of the state of their relationship with themselves rather than a statement about your value as a person, then you will, over a period of time cease to react at all." ~ Yogi Bhajan

---

There is an amazing truth here. It might be challenging to believe this for a while, because it's likely I'm a product of the world I grew up in and that means I can make anything my fault.

In this culture of right and wrong, good, and bad…it's highly likely I've learned to make myself wrong for almost anything.

Now from Yogi Bhajan's perspective I can see this all differently. I can pay attention to what he's saying here and take it in.

When someone treats me poorly, it says everything about them and nothing about me. If, however, I'm a Law of Attraction person, or just someone who learned to blame myself I will make this my fault.

My self-blame can sound like this, "Well they must be treating me this way because I haven't cleaned up my energy enough."

This isn't helpful because how do I feel when I say things like this to myself? I bet I feel bad.

What a relief it is to believe not everything is fault?

What if I can own my part in certain situations but no longer take on all the blame?

There are people that are constant projectors on this planet. They are probably not reading this book. They don't take responsibility for anything.

When I'm around someone like this, it can be very triggering and hard to unhook from, because I'm so good at taking on blame. But what if each encounter with this type of personality isn't because I've doing something wrong, or I'm not properly visualizing?

What if it's ALWAYS an opportunity to learn to let go of self-blame and to learn to accept myself exactly as I am, I little more each time?

THOUGHT FOR THE DAY: *I set the intention right now to receive whatever help needs to come to me to help shift blaming off myself.*

July 9

"As I noticed feelings and thoughts appear and disappear, it became increasingly clear that they were just coming and going on their own... There was no sense of a self-owning them."

~ Tara Brach

How wonderful is it when I learn to observe my thoughts rather than believing every thought that comes through my head? As I practice mindfulness and just notice the thoughts that just come and go, I create space between me and my thoughts. I detach more from my thoughts. I stop believing every single flipping thought that pops into my mind.

As I pay attention to my thoughts I can also notice, who is running my show? Is it my inner bully, my wounded inner child? Once I name who's running my show, while paying attention to what's being said, I detach from more of my thoughts. I take them less seriously.

I might even laugh as I notice the stream of consciousness that sounds amazingly similar to a cesspool of debilitating thoughts. That's actually magical when I laugh in the face of the inner demon. (The bully in my brain.) Then I'm able to sooth my inner child and let this part of me know she/he is okay exactly as they are no matter what the bully says. This is actually a highly effective way to quiet my bully and sooth my inner child. As this happens, I become more emotionally fit.

THOUGHT FOR THE DAY: *What if today, I can take 2-3 minutes and just notice my thoughts?*

July 10

"Your vision will become clear only when you look into your heart. Who looks outside, dreams. Who looks inside, awakens."

~ Carl Jung

This is the key to what some might call magic.

As I take the inward journey and release the learned limits that became entrenched in my being, I'm removing the clouds that block the truth of my being.

I become free of the ties that have bound me to seeing myself as a limited being.

This opens me up to possibilities far greater than the small or limited version of me can see.

With time, I trust that my needs get met in ways so much easier than all the efforting and manifesting has gotten me before.

If something doesn't seem to work out the way I think it should, I realize that it's not meant to. It's actually not for my highest good. Something better is on the horizon for me. This is likely the opposite of what I was taught. It's the opposite of what the world has taught me.

I relax more and push less, and I trust more and doubt less. Now that's magic.

THOUGHT FOR THE DAY: *What if today I can ask myself what does my heart have to tell me? Then just see what comes.*

July 11

> *"Awareness is the greatest agent for change."*
>
> *~ Eckhart Tolle*

I have often heard that awareness is the first step. This is true.

I can't shift or change what I'm unconscious too.

With tapping, I can hit a stage where I feel like I'm getting worse. The reason this can appear to be the case, is actually because more and more of my unconscious programing is becoming conscious. I see it all because my awareness has awakened.

I might appear to change a thing for a while, but I'm hyper aware of what's going on within me and around me.

If I stick with the tapping, the fever breaks. This means the flow of unconscious programing slows down.

This is why it becomes important to anchor in my wins. No matter how small they seem. As I notice and tell myself, that it's great that I'm aware, I learn to find the win in this. And it is a win. It's a big win actually.

Over time, these little wins, build a lot of momentum that's positive and my outlook becomes more positive and this builds on itself and actually creates a far more fulfilling journey of transformation.

THOUGHT FOR THE DAY*: What if today, I can notice some little wins?*

July 12

"Feelings, whether of compassion or irritation, should be welcomed, recognized, and treated on an absolutely equal basis, because both are ourselves. The tangerine I am eating is me. The mustard greens I am planting are me. I plant with all my heart and mind. I clean this teapot with the kind of attention I would have were I giving the baby Buddha or Jesus a bath. Nothing should be treated more carefully than anything else. In mindfulness, compassion, irritation, mustard green plant, and teapot are all sacred."

~ Thich Nhat Hanh

This can be a real game changer. To practice giving all of my emotions equal weight.

Then no emotion becomes forbidden. They just become emotions that come and go and come and go.

I learn to release making myself wrong for any emotion I'm experiencing.

This helps to release self-judgement. As I release more self-judgment, I take myself less seriously. I have moments when I can laugh at myself in a loving way for something in the past I might have come down on myself for.

It goes back to this, I was born with this amazing, fully loaded palette of emotions within me. Why would some be forbidden to feel, and some be acceptable to feel.

Here's my answer. They are all equal and they move through me with a lot more ease as they are felt fully.

THOUGHT FOR THE DAY: *What if all emotions are created equally?*

July 13

"As long as we have practiced neither concentration nor mindfulness, the ego takes itself for granted and remains its usual normal size, as big as the people around one will allow."

~ Ayya Khema

The ego (bully in my brain) is a producer of chaos if left unchecked.

It feeds me the worst-case scenario for every situation. It parachutes in and tells me everything I'm doing wrong.

It can sound demonic and it can be very sneaky and sound reasonable and give me all the evidence as to why it's right about me.

Here's how I tell it's the bully...

How do I feel when this voice is feeding me all the evidence as to why I should be doing better or being better? If I feel inspired (not motivated) and I'm not judging myself then I can listen to that voice, yet any "should-ing" on myself is usually fraught with bad feelings and self-judgement.

Whether I'm hearing the demon on wheels within me that's being a total ass or the reasonable, evidence-based version of this same voice, I can start to wake-up to the shit show it's feeding me and interrupt it and ask myself...

Is this the voice I want to listen too?

THOUGHT FOR THE DAY*: What if today, if I notice I'm feeling badly I can ask myself who's running my show and then ask myself is this the voice I want to listen to right now?*

July 14

"Guilt, regret, resentment, sadness & all forms of nonforgiveness are caused by too much past & not enough presence."

~ Eckhart Tolle

Forgiveness of self is so important and yet can be so dormant in my life. I may have grown up believing that somehow being hard on myself will make me change. The personal development world is filled with platitudes and pithy quotes masked as tough love but in truth just hurt me more.

If ever there was an oversight in our solar system, it's that tough love is actually a thing that's helpful.

It's not a thing. It's an oxymoron.

Love is never ever ever meant to be tough on me.

It's meant to soothe and calm me. Anyone that tells me otherwise is still asleep. That's all I need to know about them.

Anyone that uses brutal honesty and tells me they're just using tough love or just being honest with me, is also still asleep. That's all I need to know about them.

Tough love and brutal honesty are actually both just forms of hostility made to be okay when they're not.

As I sink into this truth, I wake up from the nightmare of tough love and nonforgiveness of self. As I wake up from this nightmare, I am far more capable of being more present and loving with the most important person in my life....ME.

THOUGHT FOR THE DAY: *There is no such thing as healthy tough love.*

July 15

"I do remember, and then when I try to remember, I forget."

~ Winnie the Pooh

This can be a great reminder to learn to let go of 'trying so hard.'

I live in a world that tells me all the time to try harder and push harder and be all that I can be.

What if I am all I can be right now? Right here? Forever and always.

What if I'm waking up from the belief to do more or to be more?

What if I already have everything within me? There's nothing missing or wrong with me. I just fell asleep to the truth of my being.

I can wake up and remember that I am an unlimited being, dressed in a human body. I can learn to integrate these as I allow guidance to come through me, rather than me believing I have to set goals and figure it all.

This may seem crazy or unbelievable but that's okay. What if I can just be open say…5% to the idea that there's a new way to see life and my role in it?

THOUGHT FOR THE DAY: *What if I need not figure this all out?*

July 16

---

*"The real voyage of discovery consists
not in seeking out new landscapes but in
having new eyes."*

~ Marcel Proust

Tapping and mindfulness practices both help me to see things in a new way. Especially the more I practice these techniques.

In tapping, there's a thing called a cognitive shift, which essentially means that belief changes are generated. This is having new eyes. Seeing something in a new way. Something we may have been convinced was the truth can change in a moment.

It's an amazing feature of tapping.

Mindfulness can do a similar thing with my beliefs because the more I witness my internal world and see the circus that's playing itself out in my minds, the more I question my thoughts which has the power to give me a new perspective. Once again, having new eyes.

When I see something from a new perspective, with new eyes, this creates an opening for something new to come into my experience. My life changes in front of me and I feel less edgy, less stressed, less activated. Over time this shifts so I feel peace, contentment, and fulfillment. This is the journey into awakening. One I think I might want to take.

THOUGHT FOR THE DAY: *What if today, I can tap on a circumstance, that I want to be freer around? What if the more I do this, the more I see this same circumstance from a new perspective?*

July 17

I'm here to tell you that the path to peace is right there when you want to get away.

~ Pema Chödrön

I may think that the best way to change a circumstance or a prickly person in my life is to get away from them.

This is certainly a choice I can make and yet what often seems to happen is that same circumstance shows up with a different name and different location, but the energy I feel is the same.

If I'm in a circumstance that's endangering me, I do need to act and move on from it, so I can have the space to heal more fully. If, however, a pattern keeps repeating itself in my life, then this is the perfect opportunity to heal this wound. As I tap through this pattern and how and when it shows up for me, eventually I will find I feel more peace. Then I'll find I don't seem to have this pattern showing up for me anymore, or maybe just rarely, which is good.

I can run or I can heal the wound. Either way, I get to choose what's right for me in any situation in my life.

THOUGHT FOR THE DAY: *What if today I notice a pattern that keeps rearing its head and I tap on it with the intention of just finding relief from the emotions around it. This is a great start.*

July 18

"This is the real secret of life — to be completely engaged with what you are doing in the here and now. And instead of calling it work, realize it is play."

~ Alan Watts

How wonderful this would be, yet I fall short of this often. I wonder if I'm ever this present for my life. If I'm not, I don't want to judge myself for this. I'm a product of the environment I'm living in.

I live in a world that values hard work. That reveres it even.

I bet I know a lot of hard-working people who haven't reached even a fraction of the pinnacle of success that the world puts out there as the model of success.

I would like to break free from the clutches of a culture that tells me how my life should be and what I need to look like the be considered a successful human. I want to learn to define this for myself.

I want to become so engaged with whatever I am doing that I do realize I'm having fun and not working myself to the bone. And for what?

I want to be free to do what I want so it resonates with me, independent of the opinion of others. This is true freedom if I think about it.

THOUGHT FOR THE DAY*: What if I can ask for guidance and the next right step that will lead me to a freer more enjoyable way of life? And then see what shows up.*

July 19

"Every day we are engaged in a miracle which we don't even recognize: a blue sky, white clouds, green leaves, the black, curious eyes of a child - our own two eyes. All is a miracle."

~ Thich Nhat Hanh

It's so easy to take everything for granted. That's why gratitude is a way to tune into the daily miracles that surround me.

As I drill down into the simple things in my life, like a white cloud, a bird singing, a flower, the antics of my dog or cat, I start to see how everything around me is a freaking miracle. It just takes attention (mindfulness) to notice.

The more I notice all the simple daily miracles, the more simple daily miracles I notice and the better and better I feel and the better and better my life gets.

THOUGHT FOR THE DAY: *What if today I take some time to notice the little miracles surrounding me and take them in?*

July 20

"Pure awareness transcends thinking. It allows you to step outside the chattering negative self-talk and your reactive impulses and emotions. It allows you to look at the world once again with open eyes. And when you do so, a sense of wonder and quiet contentment begins to reappear in your life."

~ Mark Williams

This is the amazing gift that tapping can produce in my life. When I tap, my brain feeds me whatever information I'm ready to see and release. Tapping also slows my mind down enough so I have access to the slower, creative part of my brain.

What is creativity but me tuning into a power greater than myself. This power does transcend thinking. It sends me messages in simple ways I formulate words for. These messages override my emotions. Yet I might get an impulse to call someone, or to email or look in a particular book. These impulses differ greatly from the reactive impulses that send me into a tizzy.

These simpler impulses are the way my authentic self speaks. I follow the impulses as I feel resonance with them, and my life unfolds in front of me rather than me pushing the agenda of my ego. It's very different way to live my life and one I will welcome the more I see how amazing it is.

THOUGHT FOR THE DAY: *What if today, I get an impulse that's inspiring and is non-reactive and I take that first step and see what comes from this?*

July 21

> *"The moment one gives close attention to anything, even a blade of grass, it becomes a mysterious, awesome, indescribably magnificent world in itself."*
>
> *~ Henry Miller*

This is mindfulness in a nutshell. Mindfulness helps me to see everyday miracles all around me.

If I look at a leaf, I notice all the little veins it has. The designs within it. The miracle it is.

If I look at my hands, I notice my fingerprints. Maybe I realize no two fingerprints are the same. I'm a unique miracle.

I see that the leaf is a world within itself. My fingerprints are a world with themselves. A bird's song is a world within itself.

I might notice how amazing my hair is, the coffee cup is, how astonishingly abundant sand is because it's millions and trillions of grains that make up a beach.

The more I start to take these daily miracles in, the more I start to realize what an amazing miracle I am and the more I find my inherent value coming into my consciousness.

THOUGHT FOR THE DAY*: What if today can be a day of everyday miracles?*

July 22

> *"In today's rush, we all think too much*
> *— seek too much — want too much — and*
> *forget about the joy of just being."*
>
> *~ Eckhart Tolle*

This might be the perfect follow up to yesterday's topic around paying closer attention to the miracles all around me.

The world I live in is a fast-paced, make it happen kind of world. It's world that measures my value by what I have, what I do and how I look.

As I awaken from this comatose programming, from thinking too much, pushing myself harder, wanting more and more, I find joy in daily life.

This joy of being can never be found in the world's view of what will make one happy. The world pushes from a very ego-driven paradigm.

It can be such a relief to stop trying so hard or needed to manifest more and more. I might see how exhausting the manifesting merry-go-round is.

I might find this simple joy of living and feel genuinely happier as I learn to let go of the world's agenda for me and walk to the beat of my own drummer.

It sounds like a better way to live.

If I find a lot of fear, doubt or resistance surfacing I can tap and find relief and then tune back into the simple things.

THOUGHT FOR THE DAY*: What if genuine well-being comes from just being more and pushing less?*

July 23

"Mindfulness, also called wise attention, helps us see what we're adding to our experiences, not only during meditation sessions but also elsewhere."

~ Sharon Salzberg

I think I like adding to my experiences. I seem to rush from one thing to next, never taking in anything fully. I run from this experience to that task. I might find I wake up and I'm already behind. So I do what the band U2 sings about. I'm running to stand still. My life just becomes a series of tasks to complete day in and day out.

I want to add to my life and all the experiences in it. And it sure seems like mindfulness gives me the chance to do just this. To take in my life moment to moment. To live more fully because I'm actually present for my life more than just rushing from one experience to the next.

I want to live more fully, breathe more deeply and even feel more fully. Mindfulness is a way to experience my life a little more every day. I like this idea a lot.

THOUGHT FOR THE DAY: *What if I can pause and take in 1- 2 minutes of mindfulness?*

July 24

"Judging is preventing us from understanding a new truth. Free yourself from the rules of old judgments and create the space for new understanding." ~ Steve Maraboli

---

What if the judgment I need to find freedom from is the judgment of self?

What if as I find freedom from judging myself, I find I need not judge others?

If I look a little closer, I think I'll find that the person I'm the hardest on and the person I judge the most relentlessly is me.

I can try not to judge others, but if I'm judging myself, I tend to judge others. It's not because I'm a bad, wrong, or a sinful person. It's because I learned to treat myself the way I was treated. Judging myself is one facet of this. So instead of telling myself that I need to stop judging others, I can start with myself and work towards self-acceptance which comes as I learn to judge myself less.

When I catch myself judging myself, I can imagine that I'm judging a small child, because that is what I am doing. I doubt I'd walk up to a little child struggling to 'be a better person' and judge them. I'd likely help them to see what's good about them. A great place to start is with the photo of myself as a child and then just try to reign judgment down on this part of me. I might do it but it's highly likely if I can, it's very painful.

I want to learn how to give myself the benefit of the doubt and tap when I find I'm being hard on myself using judgement to do it. This softens my judgment over time and then I see how I could have done nothing in my life differently. I did it exactly as I've been capable of where I was at any given moment in time. That was true then and now.

THOUGHT FOR THE DAY*: The truth if is if I could have done anything differently, I would have.*

July 25

"Suffering usually relates to wanting things to be different than they are."

~ Allan Lokos

Oh My God, I do know of this suffering. When my mind resists 'what is' I do suffer.

Any time I tell myself someone or something needs to be different for me to be okay, I suffer. The wanting things to be different is strong.

It's likely I was taught by example. Those around me had the same belief. If this or that person would just behave all would be right in the world.

251

What makes this more challenging is that I can get hundreds of people to agree with me that if this person changed their life, it would be better for everyone, yet if that person doesn't change, I suffer. It must stand to reason then that the power is within me to change me and how I see things. The truest freedom of all is to be unaffected by the insensitiveness of others. If someone can say something and I just shrug about it and don't take it on, I'm free. If I want freedom more than anything. If I'm right about something but someone else doesn't see it that way, I'm truly free if I don't need them to see I was right or see it my way.

It's journey without question and one that can take time and attention. It's also a work in progress, but a journey worth taking if I value freedom over anything else.

THOUGHT FOR THE DAY: *What if today I can ask for guidance around how to unhook from needing anything to be different than it is? Then give it some time and see what comes.*

July 26

"No one has ever been angry at another human we're only angry at our story of them.

~ Byron Katie

Gahhh!! No way. This cannot be true. I guarantee you I've been really really angry at another human. Let me count the ways and I'll give a ton of evidence as to why I should be angry at them.

To think that it's my story about them that I'm angry at is pure madness.

Trust me, I'm stark raving mad at them.

This is how tapping can save the day for me. I get to go into my anger about someone else and tap through it. I get to tap on it as much and as often as I need to. No reason to tell myself t'sf my story about them that I'm angry at. I get to allow the part of me that's committed to my anger at them have its truth about it. I get to tap and rant tap through the pure unadulterated version of my anger.

As I do this, over time, my anger at them softens. If it's someone I deal with daily I might need to tap for days or even years on the anger that can get reactivated in me again and again. This person is actually my greatest teacher; this person is revealing my wounds.

So as I keep tapping and honor my truth, eventually my truth changes. I might start to maybe, kinda, sorta, someday even agree with Bryon Katie's statement, but until that time comes, I get to tap through my truth and keep freeing myself from my anger.

THOUGHT FOR THE DAY*: As I own my anger, in its current form and tap through it, I'm doing the best thing I can for myself and ultimately for the other person, but I do it for me.*

July 27

"We cannot be present and run our
story-line at the same time."

~ Pema Chödrön

Another benefit of being more present for my life.

As I tune in to present moments and take them in more fully, I notice the noisy companions in my head seems to quiet down. My head isn't filled with the next worst thing that could go wrong, because I'm focused on the rightness of right here and right now.

The anticipatory stress that seems to run my life with fear and worry slows down and actually disappears the more present I am with what's happening in the moment.

I could use a break from all the anticipatory stress I've spent my life swimming in.

I had no idea the power of being present. I can directly experience more of the magic of being present. It's practice, like anything else I'm seeking to learn. And it's a practice that can reap astonishing rewards in my life, for my body, my mind, and my spirit.

THOUGHT FOR THE DAY: *What if today I can expand my mindfulness practice to 3-5 minutes?*

July 28

> *"Every problem perceived to be 'out there' is really nothing more than a misperception within your own thinking."*
>
> ~ Byron Katie

This might sound true in theory, but it sounds challenging in practice. I'm very used to seeing all the problems that seem to happen outside of me. I'm wired to find the problems that exist outside of me. To think that these problems are products of my misperception is a mind mess for me.

I might intellectually understand what Bryon Katie is saying as true, but I might have yet to experience this truth, because everything outside of me seems to be real. I can also get many people to agree with me. What if I can entertain the idea that whatever problem is happening outside actually started inside of my thinking. This speaks to my early imprinting. The imprinting that set my brain up to think and see from a distinct perception.

What if it's possible for my perception of things to change? And if my perceptions change, could it possible that what I experience in life changes?

It's important for me to realize, as I contemplate this idea that I have not been doing anything wrong. My life has unfolded in harmony or disharmony with my early imprinting of how life will work out. This is not my fault. If it's anything it part of a soul contract I came in with so I could evolve more fully. It will be good for me to soften self-blame. That's a big one. And I need not know how to do this. It will come over time as I release more of imprinting that caused my misperceptions in the first place. It's the journey towards emotional freedom and freedom in my way of living.

THOUGHT FOR THE DAY: *What if today I can take 2-3 minutes and tap while I tell myself, "I want to release self-blame?*

July 29

"Few of us ever live in the present. We are forever anticipating what is to come or remembering what has gone."

~ Louis L'Amour

This is true without tapping and mindfulness. Without help, I do tend to live in anticipatory stress about what might come, or I lament over what has gone and how I've wasted my life.

This is just me being mean to myself. And I can be mean to myself. I learned how to be.

Watching any child that's three years or younger, though there are always exceptions, children of this age aren't overly enculturated yet to be so mean to themselves.

They just seem to know that they are amazing and deserve every good thing. They don't know lack or lack of self-confidence yet because they are still close to the truth of their being. They haven't been programmed into full blown lack and low self-esteem. But this confidence and abundance is still in me. It's just been placed on sleep mode.

But I want can shift away from living in either anticipatory stress about what comes, or lamenting regrets from my past. As I tap through this programming and it gives way, I open up to the truest part of myself. The part that knows who I am and all that I am.

I live allowing myself to receive more good into my life and good feelings.

I need not try to get happy. Happiness comes in the moments of life when I realize I'm free to be me.

THOUGHT FOR THE DAY: *What if today I can catch myself when I'm in either living in the past or clinging to the future and interrupt my thinking?*

July 30

"The standard way of reducing stress in our culture is to put as much energy as possible into trying to arrive at a moment that matches our preferences. This ensures that we feel some level of stress until we get there (assuming we ever will) and worse, it makes the present moment into an unacceptable place to be."

~ David Cain

Words of wisdom here. To think that I may live in a constant state of the present moment being unacceptable. No wonder I feel the way I do. I can't be happy until....

What a slow death sentence.

To live believing that until I cross the finish line I've set my sights on I won't be happy.

This does make whatever is happening unacceptable for me and that's not a path I want to continue going down.

I might be understanding how mindfulness practices can help me to take in the present moment and see how much better I feel the more I practice this.

My endless bucket list becomes my presence list, which can be fulfilling.

I'd like to break free from needing to manifest my preferences and just spend more time with me in the moment and see what comes.

THOUGHT FOR THE DAY: *What if today, being in this moment can be enough?*

July 31

"Pain is not wrong. Reacting to pain as wrong initiates the trance of unworthiness. The moment we believe something is wrong, our world shrinks, and we lose ourselves in the effort to combat the pain."

~ Tara Brach

Pain is part of the human condition. It's just something that can come and go.

When I go into the pain with tapping, I help the pain to move through me, rather than locking in on the pain and telling myself I shouldn't feel this way when I do feel this way.

Owning and honoring my pain exactly where it's at in any moment is how to find genuine freedom from pain, whether the pain is mental, emotional, or physical.

As I learn to honor where I'm at in any moment, unworthiness need not enter the scene because I'm practicing worthiness through given myself the gift of my attention.

THOUGHT FOR THE DAY: *What if today I can take one step forward and let myself know that my pain is okay?*

August

August 1

---

*"We must be willing to encounter
darkness and despair when they come up
and face them, over and over again if need
be, without running away or numbing
ourselves in the thousands of ways we
conjure up to avoid the unavoidable."*

~ *Jon Kabat-Zinn*

This might sound like a scary proposition for me if I've been enculturated to believe that I shouldn't feel, or that I should limit what, when, and how I feel. Sigmund Freud says it this way, "Unexpressed emotions will never die. They are buried alive and will come forth later in uglier ways."

I need not swan dive into expressing my emotions fully, but I can take baby steps to do this. Tapping is a highly effective way to allow me to go into the depths of my suppressed emotions to feel and then release them. If I feel afraid to do this, I can start right here and tap through the fact that I am afraid to feel fully. I meet myself where I'm at with tapping and honor each step that comes up for me.

I need not push myself to feel or push myself to "get through this." I start with honoring my personal journey through what can appear to be a minefield.

I can tap on the anticipatory stress I feel about going deeper into my emotional landscape. This is a way to ease into and opening up to feeling more fully.

With tapping, when I experience strong emotions, I know this is a good sign because it's letting me know that I've targeted some repressed energy coming up, and I can remind myself this is a good thing. It's letting me know that emotional energy is being released from my body and over time, or maybe even immediately, I will feel lighter and freer. This is evidence that I'm releasing this cellular debris from my body.

This allows the mind-body healing to begin, and this is what's on the other side of going deeper into my emotions and releasing them. It's a huge win.

THOUGHT FOR THE DAY*: What if today I can just consider that going into the depths of my emotions with support has the power to change my life for the better? I'm just considering this.*

August 2

"We do so much, we run so quickly, the situation is difficult, and many people say, "Don't just sit there, do something." But doing more things may make the situation worse. So you should say, "Don't just do something, sit there." Sit there, stop, be yourself first, and begin from there.

~ Thich Nhat Hanh

This is counter-intuitive to the high octane, fast-paced, make-it-happen world I live in. Let me get this straight. Instead of trying harder and pushing more, I'm supposed to sit back and relax instead? I might be asking, "How is anything going to get done?" This might even blow my mind and feel uncomfortable because it goes against everything I've been taught to believe. But what if it is possible that the ducks are flying in the wrong direction? What if the loudest voice, the most prominent voice isn't the truest voice?

As I relax more, I soothe my nervous system and lower cortisol levels (the stress hormone), and as I do this, I now have access to the prefrontal cortex, the less reactive, critical thinking part of the brain. This part of my brain has access to solutions I just can't see when I'm all revved up on stress energy. When I'm relaxed, helpful things just come because my prefrontal cortex has room to think.

Even if I set aside what might sound like spiritual mumbo jumbo, it does make sense that calming down and stepping away from a problem can bring me the solution when I'm, say, taking a shower. Hmm! No wonder great ideas can come while I'm in the shower. I'm generally more relaxed and calm.

So I can believe in forces at work that have my back, or I can set that aside and see I have access to the more creative, problem-solving part of my brain when I relax more and stress less.

THOUGHT FOR THE DAY*: What if I can step away from a problem or challenge today and come back to it later and see if a solution comes to me? It's worth trying.*

August 3

"Stepping out of the busyness, stopping our endless pursuit of getting somewhere else, is perhaps the most beautiful offering we can make to our spirit."

~ Tara Brach

This may sound amazing. If it does, my soul resonates with this truth. If I feel uncomfortable with this idea, that lets me know my ego (the inner bully) is in charge. The bully fills my inner child with fear. It wants my child self to believe that danger is always lurking around the corner.

The bully is just that, a bully. It's like the schoolyard punk who masks fear with bravado and domination. It beats up on the child who wears their fear on their sleeve. There's no bravado available for my inner child.

And thus, the inner battle begins.

As I pause and tune in and I realize that I don't want either of these inner characters taking the lead in life or deciding for me, my healthy adult self or authentic self gets put back in charge. As I calm down, my decision-making capabilities return and the decisions I make are no longer made from fear.

As Tosha Silver states, "Decisions get made through me rather than by me." This is a far more balanced and peaceful way to live. It's a way that's not taught in this high-octane world, but as I practice distancing myself from all the pushing the world pushes on me like a dope dealer, I see there is another way. There is a better way.

I realize that I'm not intended to push and manifest my way through life. I open up to greater awareness and more fruitful possibilities that feel good and fuel inspiration. Then I realize this is the way I've always been meant to live.

THOUGHT FOR THE DAY: *What if today, when I catch myself in pushing mode, I can just take a moment and step back? What if this pause is enough for today?*

August 4

"Our own self-love draws a thick veil between us and our faults." ~ Lord Chesterfield

Learning to love ourselves is its own journey. It starts with self-acceptance. As I learn to make my flawed behavior okay, I practice self-acceptance. As I learn to make all of my emotions okay to feel, I practice self-acceptance. As I learn to rest when I feel the need to rest instead of pushing through, I'm honoring my needs. As I learn to send loving kindness to all the wounded parts of me, I practice self-love.

Each day I can practice being mindful of my internal world but asking myself,

"Who's running my show? Do I want to listen with the part of me that's running my show, or do I want to dispel what it's feeding me, if it's not in my best interest?"

As I attend to whatever is presenting itself in my life in moments of presence, I am practicing self-love. As I learn to make whatever is happening okay in any moment, I find more self-acceptance coming from within me and more self-love that comes through the practice of self-acceptance.

This chips away at the "wrongness of me" that I've learned.

Anything that I'm doing that appears not to be serving me is really a way I'm trying to protect myself. Anything that I'm not doing that would serve me better is still a way I'm trying to protect myself from the unknown.

Anyway I slice it, I'm always trying to help myself in a way that can be misguided, but it's still me trying to protect me. As I learn to see this truth, the self-judgment that's reigned its fear down on me finds its way through me.

On the other side of this is a more self-accepting, self-loving me. The me I've always been meant to be.

THOUGHT FOR THE DAY: *What if today I tell myself that I'm okay exactly as I am right now?*

August 5

"Look at other people and ask yourself if you are really seeing them or just your thoughts about them."

~ Jon Kabat-Zinn

This can be mind blowing. What I find, if I suspend judgment, can be that I am witnessing thoughts I have about someone. I'm telling a story in my mind about them.

Now, I might have a lot of evidence to prove that my thoughts are accurate, but if I didn't have this history, or these thoughts about them, then I might have a different perception of them.

Here's another way of saying this: If I'd bet money that someone was going to behavior a certain way, this is showing my perception of them. It's far more likely that someone will behave according to my historical perception of them.

It can be an interesting experiment to try. If I interrupt my thoughts about someone, that I'd bet money would behave a certain way, I might just shift my energy (my story) about them, and then see if things can change.

A great way to do this is to tap through my current "truth" around them until I find relief. As I keep doing this, I might find I see them in a new way. If this happens, and I'm feel free of my past with them, I might notice little differences that can be indications that the energy between us is now different because I'm different about it.

Again, it can just be a way to experiment if I'm up for it. If it brings me some peace, then it would be worth it. Since the only true freedom I have comes from within me, this could be a powerful practice.

THOUGHT FOR THE DAY*: What if today I can pick a person, or a circumstance, and tap through my truth and see if I just notice a feeling of relief? Then see what happens.*

August 6

"We often have very little empathy for our own thoughts and feelings and frequently try to suppress them by dismissing them as weaknesses."

~ Mark Williams

Weakness. This is such a prevalent word in the world of the bully in my brain, especially with emotions. It's been said that someone is strong for not feeling fully, but this couldn't be further from the truth. Anyone that's walked the journey of feeling fully knows that feeling deeply is a courageous act, even more so if I come from a culture that tells me I'm strong for keeping a stiff upper lips or putting my big girl or big boy pants on.

When I don't feel fully, I don't create genuine empathy for my thoughts and feelings. I'm too busy suppressing my emotions. I'm rating myself as strong because I didn't let my feelings "get the best of me."

Anyone that has allowed themselves the true depth of their grief knows the courage this takes. Anyone who has dealt with a betrayal knows the depths of their feelings. Anyone who goes deeply into any emotion knows the courage this takes.

Someone may appear to "have their shit together" because they don't feel, but at what cost? Most of the time this cost remains hidden until it can't hide any more.

If I've tapped before now, it's likely that I know what it's like to feel fully. It might feel intense until the intensity gives way to a lightness meant to be. My emotional load lightens, and life becomes more manageable and, dare I say, even more enjoyable.

THOUGHT FOR THE DAY: *What if feeling fully sets me free and brings out the lightness within me?*

August 7

---

*"Acknowledging the pain and the
suffering that take place inside you, and
allowing the feelings, will take time, but this
new way of handling these feelings will
change the way you relate to you and to the
outside world."*

~ Kelly Martin

This is a true possibility for me. As I acknowledge my pain and suffering and give it a much-needed voice, and use tapping to help me release the pain and suffering, I do find I become more emotional fit and more emotional available for myself. As I do this, I might find I look outside of myself less and less for validation. I'm giving to myself what I need most. If someone else validates and support me, that just becomes icing on top of the cake.

It's such an ironic thing. As I learn to give to myself what I've tried to get from others, I end up receiving from others as well. I receive from others because I am free. I open up the space to receive because I'm no longer groping for someone else to meet my needs. This is the truest freedom of all, and yet one not often taught.

THOUGHT FOR THE DAY: *What if I can just contemplate that I'm meant to be free in this way?*

August 8

"*You are not a drop in the ocean. You are the entire ocean, in a drop.*" ~ *Rumi*

I might be wondering what this even means. Depending on how I grew up, I may have a lot of learned limits around the idea that I am so much more than I've ever been taught to believe. I might have told that I'm born unworthy, born sinful, born needing redemption. How could an innocent infant come into the world born in need of these things?

This is the teachings of a culture based heavily in ego consciousness. This is also the sound of the bully in my brain.

What if the opposite is true of me? What if, like Rumi says, I'm not just a drop in the ocean? What if within me exists an entire ocean of possibilities I haven't even tuned into? What if this could be true?

THOUGHT FOR THE DAY: *I can start by carrying this thought with me today… What if there is an ocean of possibility within me I can tune into?*

271

August 9

"You are imperfect, permanently and inevitably flawed. And you are beautiful. "

~ Amy Bloom

If I could embrace the last part of this truth where it says, "And you are beautiful," I'd probably feel better about myself.

Maybe it feels impossible to agree that, despite my imperfections, and despite me being permanently and inevitably flawed, as a human I am beautiful. That part I might struggle with. What if I can learn to believe that I'm beautiful, flaws, foibles, and all? I need not use affirmations to get me to believe this. They won't work if my brain puts up a fight. Right now my brain might not say that I'm beautiful and agree. There's a simple but effective way to work with this.

Let me bridge this, meaning let me add in words to soften the statement so my brain can believe it:

"What if overtime I can learn to believe that even though, as humans, I'm not perfect and I have certain flaws, there is beauty in me anyway?"

Can my brain believe this, more than the original statement? If it does, then I'm moving in the right direction. I can keep building from here.

Let me try another version:

"I may be imperfect. I may have flaws, but what if the beauty really is in the imperfections?"

I can play with any statement and reword it so my brain agrees. I like that I can believe more good things about me using bridging statements to do it.

THOUGHT FOR THE DAY: *What if today I can take one affirmation and rewrite it so my brain believes it? Even if just a little bit, this is progress.*

August 10

"Because one believes in oneself, one doesn't try to convince others. Because one is content with oneself, one doesn't need others' approval. Because one accepts oneself, the whole world accepts him or her."

— *Lao Tzu*

Wow! That sounds amazing on one level, but I might be nowhere near this. Like not even in the same solar system.

What if that's okay? What if this is just revealing that some wounds need some attention? What's important to remember is that no one feels this way all the time.

Some days I'm more confident than others. Some days I'm more centered than others. Some days I can laugh at myself and my imperfections. On other days... not so much. I might spiral down into an abyss of self-loathing.

On days like these, tapping and mindfulness are highly effective tools to help me find relief from that insane bully in my brain always feeding me fear. As I learn to recognize and tap through this part of me, it does loosen its grip on me.

This is all I need to look for. Relief from these worrisome, fear-based thoughts that send me down the rabbit hole of worst-case scenarios. The more mindful I become of this inner bully and tap, the less potent and less true whatever it's feeding me feels.

THOUGHT FOR THE DAY*: What if today if I catch myself heading down the rabbit hole of fear, I can use tapping just to find relief?*

August 11

"You can search throughout the entire universe for someone who is more deserving of your love and affection than you are yourself, and that person is not to be found anywhere. You, yourself, as much as anybody in the entire universe, deserve your love and affection. "
~ Sharon Salzberg

Oh to love myself more. What if this is possible? What if this starts with practicing self-acceptance? What if self-love is a practice?

I didn't learn to feel badly about myself in an instant. There was consistent programming going on that was fed to me. This trained my brain to see myself from a less loving and less kind place. As I interrupt the less than loving, unkind thinking that goes on between my ears, I'll feel better naturally, without having to try to.

THOUGHT FOR THE DAY: *What if today I can practice (even if I don't believe it yet) telling myself I'm okay, no matter what the bully says?*

August 12

"You have peace," the old woman said,
"when you make it with yourself."

~ Mitch Albom

Sounds great, but how do I do this?

Tapping allows me my fully loaded, unadulterated truth, in a safe and healthy way. I might find it hard to give my truth to myself, but with support and with practice I can learn to tap and tell my truth for myself. I need not go to someone and spew all over them. I can do this by tapping and using it to find relief.

Peace isn't something I have to find or seek. Trying to find inner peace is like putting a band-aid on a broken limb. Peace can well up from within me as I attend to the learned limits that have been a big part of my experience.

Peace is a by-product of allowing myself my truth while using tapping to acknowledge and honor myself. As I find a safe and healthy way for myself to express my truth, peace comes with ease because I've released what's blocking the peace that's already in me.

THOUGHT FOR THE DAY: *What if today I can remind myself that, as I allow myself my truth, peace comes from within me?*

August 13

"Live your life, sing your song. Not full of expectations. Not for the ovations. But for the joy of it."

~ Rasheed Ogunlaru

I want to learn how to do this. I love the sound of this. To live my life without it being full of expectations. What a relief.

The world I live in loves expectations. It loves telling me to make it happen and to keep pushing. It tells me to compete, and be the best version of myself, as if that's not already in me. It teaches me to seek ovations from others. The world I live in teaches all about winners and losers. I want to break free from this madness.

I want to believe there is no such thing as competition when I'm in touch with my authentic self. There is no need to push and pressure myself because life can unfold in amazing ways when I stop the pushing.

To live my life for the joy of living it may feel impossible in a world that tells me who I should be, what I should do, and how I should look. But I have heard about people who have chucked away the trappings of the ego and the material world and lived their truth. They've dropped all convention and lived true to themselves.

What if this can be me too? What if I can continue to attend to the learned limits I've adopted and, as these fall away, I find my authentic self has been patiently waiting to greet me again?

THOUGHT FOR THE DAY: *What would it take for me to live in a way that's true for me? I need not uproot my life. I need not scare myself, but I can just contemplate this and see what next step might be revealed.*

August 14

---

*How you love yourself is how you teach
others to love you.*

~ Rupi Kaur

This one can really get to me. This seems to add insult to injury. Once again, there's something else that's my fault. To be honest, I'm tired of blaming myself for anything and everything.

If others don't treat me well, to tell myself that it's because I don't love myself just dishes out more self-blame.

How about this: If others don't treat me well, it's because I learned to treat myself the way I was treated. I might have a hard time being loving to myself if this wasn't modeled towards me.

If I'd been given all the loving sentiments and had been told I was worthy and wonderful, I would know how to love myself because it was shown to me. This is exactly why it takes practice to learn how to love myself. And it's likely I will bump up against non-loving individuals in my life, not because I'm bad, wrong, or unlovable, but to show me the wounding I have around this.

This is a much better way to see this. The unloving people in my life are my greatest teachers. I may not like this yet, but it's true, and at least I'm not drowning in more blame.

THOUGHT FOR THE DAY: *It's not my fault I don't love myself well, but I can learn how to love myself more fully.*

August 15

"I laugh at myself. I don't take myself completely seriously. I think that's another quality that people have to hold on to... you have to laugh, especially at yourself."

~ Madonna

If I have a lot of expectations for myself, it's likely I might have a hard time laughing at myself. This is okay. It's not like I can flip some imaginary switch and suddenly not take myself so seriously.

I can notice the part of me that takes it all really seriously. The part of me that puts me in the pressure cooker all the time. There's no room for humor in a pressure cooker.

What if this is a great place to start? Just to notice all the pressure I've been under. Noticing is the best first step.

As I notice, I detach even just a little from the pressurized part of me. The part that pushes and never lets up. The "just one more thing" part of me. This is the bully in my brain that pushes and fills me with fear if I'm not always producing. This is the doer part of me that can be relentless, especially if it's not balanced with quiet moments to allow inspiration to come.

As I learn to allow inspiration to come through me, I bet I find more peace and acceptance and maybe even laughter that includes not taking myself so seriously because I've softened the beliefs that I am what I do and I am what I have. Then I stop pushing myself so hard, so there's room to laugh and be free.

THOUGHT FOR THE DAY*: What if today I can ask for just a step to be revealed to me as to how to pressurize myself less so I can laugh a little more?*

August 16

"It is not worth the while to let our imperfections disturb us always."

~ Henry David Thoreau

I would agree with Thoreau, and yet I'm not sure how to do this. How do I get to the place where my imperfections disturb me less than they might now?

I own them. How do I own them?

Tapping helps me to own my truth. Tapping allows my mind to feed me whatever information I am ready to face about myself so I can be free of its grip. As I tap and tell the story of any person or circumstance that does disturb me, I own it, and in owning this I find relief from it. This helps me to see these exact same people and circumstances in a new way.

I gain new perspectives that help me to feel freer. I gain new understanding I didn't have before. I learn to let my imperfections just be one part of me rather than my whole story. They're just aspects of me. They are not the whole of who I am.

The irony is, the more I own my imperfections and face them, the less they disturb me and the better I feel about myself.

THOUGHT FOR THE DAY: *What if today I can pick one imperfection and simply remind myself this trait, this characteristic, is just one small part of me?*

August 17

"I now see how owning our story and loving ourselves through that process is the bravest thing that we will ever do."

~ Brené Brown

Imagine owning my full story. If someone looked in the window of my life when I was child, what might they feel for me? As I learn to embrace the fullness that is me, I own all aspects of me. The good, the bad, the ugly, and the beautiful. These are part of what makes me, me. Any emotional scars I have are part of what makes me, me.

Allowing myself to walk through the fire of my history and use tapping to put my history where it belongs—in the past—is very brave.

I'm in a body, subject to the full palette of emotions I came installed with. Emotions meant to be felt through to their completion. As I learn to do this, my past no longer haunts me. It is a part of me, but the emotional charges buried in my body get released. This helps me to find more emotional freedom.

I live well. I live a good life. I experience happiness and so much more. I want to believe this is true for me. This happens as I learn to free myself from the emotional ties that have bound me up and had me living a narrower version of my life. As I own my life story and own everything that's made me, me, I find freedom and liberation on the other side. I like that freedom and liberation can be mine.

THOUGHT FOR THE DAY: *What if today I can consider that owning my story and feeling fully can set me free?*

August 18

"If you begin to understand what you are without trying to change it, then what you are undergoing is a transformation."

~ Jiddu Krishnamurti

Sounds like more acceptance. This is a cornerstone of healing and emotional freedom. To understand that I am a multifaceted being is a great beginning. I'm not a black and white photo. I have many aspects and many colors to who I am as this human. Every single aspect, character trait, and all of my supposed flaws make up exactly who I am right now.

The parts of me I have learned to believe aren't acceptable are the very parts of me that need my love. I may have been taught to reject the less than perfect parts of me, but these less than perfect parts are my greatest teachers. These are my wounded parts, and these wounds, despite some teachings, are not my fault.

Call them soul contracts. Call them divinely orchestrated experiences, but what if the roughest parts of me, the worried parts of me, the seeming less desirable parts of me, are the parts with the power to teach me all about genuine self-love.

Whether I'm a bible user or not, in the King James version of the Bible, Jesus was quoted as saying, "But I say unto you, love your enemies, bless them that curse you, do good to them that hate you, and pray for them which despitefully use you, and persecute you." This is tall order for even the most illuminated among us, but what if this starts with how I treat myself. What if I can learn to love the enemy parts within myself? What if I can learn to bless myself despite the ways I've learned to curse, persecute, and hate myself? What if I can ask for help from my authentic self to learn how to love all of me?

This can take root within me. It can be like any seed. It can grow and bloom into fuller and freer love of myself exactly as I am right here, right now. I think I'm meant to feel good about myself. I think I'm meant to release the learned limits that have shackled me to self-recrimination. I think I would like to start today with a love affair with myself.

THOUGHT FOR THE DAY*: I may not know how, but I like that I can be guided as to the how of this.*

August 19

"The mistake ninety-nine percent of humanity made, as far as Fats could see, was being ashamed of what they were; lying about it, trying to be somebody else."

~ J.K. Rowling, The Casual Vacancy

Whoa! Could this be another self-acceptance, bordering on self-love reminder? I think so. So far, I've probably lived my life-giving lip service to loving myself. The truth might be that I don't have a clue as to how to do this. Do I just say all kinds of loving affirmations to myself? Maybe. If this resonates with me, yes.

What if I need not know the how? I need not figure this out. What if I just open up a little more today to the idea that the "how" can be shown? What if it's important to learn to practice self-love? What if self-love springs up from within me as I practice releasing the muck of learned limits that I've unconsciously adopted over the years?

In this way, self-love becomes something that does bubble up from within me. It's not something "out there" that I need to pull into me. It's already in me. It just needs some space to shine through me. I like this idea a lot. It saves me from the endless, exhausting pursuit of self-love.

THOUGHT FOR THE DAY: *What if today I can take 2-3 minutes and just sit and do nothing and see what surfaces for me? What if this is a way to be present with the most important person in my life, me?*

August 20

"Stop trying to be less of who you are.
Let this time in your life cut you open and
drain all of the things that are holding you
back."

~ Jennifer Elisabeth

In this world with a cookie cutter mentality of needing to fit in while simultaneously standing out and being different, things can feel daunting. My inner child self will either sell her/his soul to be a part of my tribe and fit in, or it might rail against it. Either way, it's the opposite end of the same spectrum.

What if I was never meant to fit in? What if I've always been meant to be unabashedly me? This can feel unsafe for me though and this makes sense. If I grew up in a system that wants power and control over me then to draw outside the lines of this system can be threatening for me.

What if there are others like me that want to be supported in giving fullness to their authentic selves? What if this is another thing I need not figure out?

If I'm someone who hasn't felt a lot of trust in others, that's okay. What if I can ask for guidance to help me learn to trust? This is a way I can practice opening up to receiving answers. I can remain filled with doubt but ask anyway. My asking can sound something like this:

"I am filled with doubt. I am filled with mistrust. I want to believe, but I don't. I want to believe that I am meant to live true to myself. I want to be free of the need to fit in or to defy, but I don't know how to be free. I want to open to trust and faith. If I'm meant to be someone who has faith and trust, then show me the way. Open me up and drain me of what's in my way. This is my best right now."

My asking need not be flowery, pretty, or well stated. If authentically and imperfectly asked for, this is enough.

THOUGHT FOR THE DAY*: What if I can ask to be opened up? What if this is enough?*

August 21

"When you stop living your life based on what others think of you real life begins. At that moment, you will finally see the door of self-acceptance opened."

~ Shannon L. Alder

Learning to let go of the need for approving others is its own journey. Yesterday, I was shown the idea of asking for guidance. I can tap to help me to open up and drain what is in my way. Tapping allows me to access what's in my way without having to figure it out. With tapping, learned limits get revealed, and drained.

The need for approval is a survival tactic of my inner child. If a child feels that it won't be approved of, they fear banishment from their tribe. When my inner child fears rejection or banishments, this part of me will do anything to be brought back into the fold. This part of me is all about surviving and my inner child is brilliant because she/he figured out how to survive on their own. What if I can give my inner child credit for this? This is the way I learned to survive—by fitting in or defying.

Now I may be ready to begin the journey of living, so it feels more congruent with my authentic self. I might be feeling that inner pull to take a new step in a new direction. I need not do anything that freaks me out right now, but I can continue the inner journey of clearing and opening. This is more than enough because, as I continue to do this, a way becomes clear step by step.

THOUGHT FOR THE DAY: *What if today I can just take another simple step forward and tap on something that feels like a block and see what happens?*

August 22

---

*"We are at our most powerful the
moment we no longer need to be powerful."*

~ Eric Micha'el Leventhal

Pursuing power is an endless journey down the rabbit hole of the ego striving for more. Pursuing more can be exhausting. The world tells me to keep pursuing more, but the challenge is this is outwardly focused. The inner journey gets ignored and this is a high price to pay.

I may have heard of some "successful" people who have reached what some might believe is the pinnacle of success, and they talk about how it's not fulfilling. Some of these successful people have even taken their own lives. They appear to "have it all," and yet it's clear this success is not fulfilling for them.

The pushing of the world to pursue success is so loud and so strong that I can still overlook the misery still within many successful people. This is because the world I live in defines success by the money in my bank account, the car I drive, and the house I live in. If I don't have these things, or have less than what is considered successful, I can feel bad about myself.

But does The Great Spirit that runs all really push this agenda, or is this the ego's agenda? It's a good thing to go within and see what answer comes back. It's the quiet voice that carries truth within it. It's not the voice filled with bravado and pounding its chest. That's the voice of the world; the voice that competes and tries to be a winner.

I want to hear the voice of my soul. The voice of my authentic self. This voice is calm and carries peace for me with it. I want to learn to follow the voice that brings me peace.

THOUGHT FOR THE DAY: *What if today, when I hear the loud voice of the world, I can just pause and go within just for a moment?*

August 23

*"Commandment #1: Believe in yourself.
Commandment #2: Get over yourself."*

~ Kristan Higgins

Let me break this down.

Believe in yourself. Nice sentiment, but how? How does one just believe in themselves?

Oh, and I love the follow-up to this. "Get over yourself." Sounds suspiciously like the sneakier side of the bully in my brain, all dressed up in personal development jargon. I want to divorce myself from anything that judges me and tells me to just get over myself. I've done that to myself for a long time now.

Believing in myself can come through tapping and mindfulness practices. To just tell me to believe in myself isn't enough. That's like telling me to just stop worrying or to just put the fork down. I can pray for a miracle for sure, but meanwhile I can tap to release what's keeping me from remembering the truth of my being and believing in myself. As I do this, believing myself comes naturally through.

Getting over myself is punitive. I would like to believe that I need not get over myself. I can learn to get into myself more and see the fully loaded human and spiritual being I am.

THOUGHT FOR THE DAY*: What if today I can go into myself rather than get over myself and get a closer look at what's going on within me?*

August 24

"What would happen if you stopped fighting, and gave yourself permission to feel? Not just the good things, but everything?"

~ R.J. Anderson

What would happen if I laid down the sword passed on to me in a world that avoids feeling fully? What if there was not a single emotion that was forbidden to me, no matter what it was? This is the basis for the book *Forbidden Emotions - The Key to Healing.*

I am encouraged to go down deeper into all of my emotions so I can feel them and be set free. The caveat is I can use tapping to help me feel more fully and release the emotions stored in my body.

In neuroscience, the body is the subconscious mind. My body is actually an amazing companion. It carries the unexpressed emotions I've buried for a long time. I am encouraged to feel everything in a safe and healthy way for me, using tapping to do so, because as I do this, I release my body of the stuck emotions and I free my body and mind so my spirit now can come through.

When I feel even my darkest of emotions with the support I need, I release what I got wired backwards in the feelings arena. To not feel fully is to suppress. As these emotions build up inside of me, they have to go somewhere eventually, and they usually do in ways that seem explosive or over the top. I might do and say things that hurt someone else.

It's important to know that it's never the emotions that are the problem. It's the actions that come from suppressing emotions that are the problem. This is an incentive to feel more fully because I become emotionally balanced the more I allow my emotions their fuller expression. I'm less likely to behave in ways I later regret.

THOUGHT FOR THE DAY: As I learn to feel fully, I release stuck emotions from my body. Over time, I become far more emotionally fit and able to respond rather than react.

August 25

"No tree tries to become a certain kind of tree. No flower tries to become a certain kind of flower. The tree and the flower open up to the sun and soak up water. Thus, they grow into themselves. No judgment. No expectations. No commentary. Your task is the same. If you can stop trying so hard to become who you think you should be, and instead commit to understanding and nourishing yourself, you will bloom into whatever kind of person you are." ~

Vironika Tugaleva

In much of the personal development world, I am encouraged to become the best version of myself. To be all I can be. To just do it. To get over myself. To commit to Constant and Never-Ending Improvement (CANEI). Sounds exhausting.

What I might not know is that the personal development world is very ego based, and thus pushes this agenda. It's my fault if things in my life aren't changing. I must not be trying hard enough. I must not be tuning into my vision board daily. I must once again be doing something wrong. This only elevates anxiety and lowers my self-esteem simultaneously (as if I need more of either of these).

What if, as Vironika states here, I can see this all differently? What if I can actually stop all the "trying" so hard? This may feel uncomfortable at first because it goes against many things I've been taught, but it is a journey worth taking.

I know there are other people out there right now who are feeling just like me. What if I start to magically meet these people as I unhook from the world of the ego? What if the journey opens me up to greater possibilities than I've known before? I get to decide now which path I want to take. The pushing and trying path, or the opening and allowing path.

THOUGHT FOR THE DAY: *What if today I can look at advertising and ask myself, "What are they trying to sell me?" This is a great place to unhook from the world of the ego.*

August 26

"Self-esteem is the reputation we acquire with ourselves."

~ *Nathaniel Branden*

I don't think I've ever thought about it this way. The relationship I cultivate with myself is what grounds me in who I am.

Now, I can do this from the pushing, trying perspective and try to be all I can be, or I can cultivate a relationship with whatever I believe is a power greater than my human self and see what might happen. If I take the latter path, I bet I will find that my life opens up in ways I never thought were possible before.

What if all the struggles and exhaustion I've been feeling for a while now is how this power greater than my human self has been trying to get my attention and guide me to a new way of living? What if as I practice and cultivate this new way of being, of asking for guidance and then stepping back and allowing, even just a little bit, I am surprised at what unfolds for me?

I notice synchronicities that come to me that I feel inspired to act on. I might even throw out my list of goals, so I create more space for things to come to me that are better than my goal list has in store for me.

This is all counterintuitive to what the world sells me, but I can be reminded that maybe the majority of the ducks are flying in the wrong direction. And like Robert Frost once talked about, I take the road less traveled, and this does make all the difference.

THOUGHT FOR THE DAY: *What if today, when I have a decision to make, I ask myself, "Which road feels right and true for me, regardless of popular opinion?*

August 27

"At the end of the day, remind yourself that you did the best you could today, and that is good enough.""

~ Lori Deschene

What a relief this can be. It's also possible that I will feel uncomfortable doing this at first.

If I've had an epic, unmanaged bully in the brain that's constantly feeding me fear and worry, then this can be a hump to get over. Both tapping and mindfulness are great practices to help me manage my inner bully and find relief so I can take steps forward towards this practice.

I can start by telling myself that I've done the best I could today and then notice the "yeah, but's" that surface.

"I did the best I could today." "Yeah, but you should have done this better."

I did the best I could today." "Yeah, but you shouldn't have said that to them."

"I did the best I could today." "Yeah, but you know better and you did that anyway."

Even reading these three examples can be exhausting.

The bully in my brain is on the relentless pursuit to fill me with fear, worry, and missing out. With tapping, I can tap through whatever follows my "yeah, buts" and soften the grip the bully has on me. I can also use mindfulness to pay attention to who is running my inner show and then question whether or not this is the voice I want to listen to today.

As I practice either of these, I will find the bully quiets down and not occupy so much of my head space. As it quiets more, I will find that better thoughts occupy my head, and I do believe that I have done the best I can for today. Believing the good is evidence that I'm changing my physiology for the better. This is a big win.

THOUGHT FOR THE DAY*: What if tonight I can tell myself that I am doing the best I can and that I will believe this is true over time?*

August 28

> "The most adventurous journey to embark on; is the journey to yourself, the most exciting thing to discover; is who you really are, the most treasured pieces that you can find; are all the pieces of you, the most special portrait you can recognize; is the portrait of your soul."
>
> ~ C. JoyBell

What if the portrait of my soul is in me, and it's patiently waiting for me to recognize this? What if guidance is always available to me, I just can't see it or hear it because the voice of the world I live in promotes the voice of my ego (the bully in my brain)?

What if, as I soften the haunting effects my inner bully has on me, I actually recognize my soul's voice is always there for me? I recognize that I have done nothing wrong, I just got programmed to believe something very different than the truth of my being.

As C. Joybell states, this is a journey back to connecting to my soul, or my authentic self. It's not a straight or linear line. It can come and go as I shake off the voice of the world I live in that is deeply rooted in the ego-consciousness. I can think about it this way. I'm on a journey out of the darkness of the world's view to a lightness that is my true self. It's just like waking up from a nightmare. I might have to shake things off for a while, but eventually I land back to communion with my authentic self. The journey back to my authentic self is worth taking.

THOUGHT FOR THE DAY*: What if my authentic self is always available? I can learn how to tune into this part of me.*

August 29

---

*"No amount of self-improvement can
make up for any lack of self-acceptance."*

~ *Robert Holden*

This is healing in a nutshell; acceptance of myself.

This also makes sense as to why I may have tried many self-improvement programs with limited results. If my self-concept is not addressed, I can be given every practical step to take, take the steps perfectly, and still not see results.

This means that the emotional part of me needs attention. If I haven't learned to believe that every single emotion I have is acceptable, then I won't have self-acceptance. Without self-acceptance I can make myself wrong for anything and everything. The bully in my brain loves to help me see all the ways I'm wrong and unacceptable.

As I use tapping to free myself from a lack of self-acceptance, I feel that I am acceptable exactly as I am. I even have those amazing moments when I laugh at myself in the best way.

Mindfulness practices, like noticing when the bully is feeding me evidence as to why I am unacceptable and then questioning these thoughts, are simple ways to release the story around how unacceptable I am. In this way, I make space for the truth of my being to come shining through. This has all the evidence as to how acceptable I really am and actually always have been.

THOUGHT FOR THE DAY*: What if today, if I catch myself thinking I need to improve this or that, I can pause and let myself know that even with this I am acceptable? I don't even have to believe this yet.*

August 30

"Something, somewhere, knows what's best for me and promises to keep sending me people and experiences to light my way as long as I live in gratitude and keep paying attention to the signs. "

~ Jennifer Elisabeth

This is my soul, my authentic self, the true self, a Force of good, The Great Spirit, The Universe, Source, God that knows what's best for me. That constantly sends me winks, impulses to take inspired action and lays out breadcrumbs for me to follow.

The challenge is the noise of the world always shouting from the rooftops and sending advertising to convince me my life will be so much better if possess or do this next thing.

The noise of the world is a formidable foe. Releasing this programming is the journey of a lifetime.

This journey actually just requires that I question the thoughts that fire off in my mind all the time. The constant stream of thoughts that's like a ticker tape going on and on.

The more I question my thoughts, the less I believe them. The less I believe them, the more I notice the guidance is always available and the more I turn away from the loud voice of the world and towards the voice that comes from within me.

As I live more from a place of gratitude about all the little things here for me, I get a clearer signal because I'm tuning into the gratitude all around me and the voice of spirit calling me back home to my true self.

THOUGHT FOR THE DAY: *What if today I can take 2-3 minutes and just get quiet with no agenda?*

August 31

---

*"Don't let others box you into their idea
of what they think you should be. A
confined identity is a miserable way to exist.
Be you and live free. Trust that in living true
to yourself, you will attract people that
support and love you, just as you are."*

~ Jaeda DeWalt

This is the "why" for why I should question my thoughts and tune into who's running my show. As I do this, I recognize the voice of the world around me that speaks in shoulds and need to's and have to's. As I continue to unhook from this programming, I will notice that I'm naturally living true to myself. It's not something I have to push or try for, it just is.

I free myself from the constraints placed on me in a world that teaches fitting in rather than being free. I break out of the box of learned limits and feel lighter and freer and notice more grace and ease in my life.

The journey to this place is often through my emotions and the acceptance of them. As I walk this path, I find I am living truer to myself than ever before, and I do find people showing up in my life who love and support this in me. They can do this because they, too, are walking this path back to their authentic self.

We meet in that field of common good.

THOUGHT FOR THE DAY*: What if today I can just notice the places I'm feeling confined? I need not do anything right now other than just notice.*

September

September 1

> *"No negative thoughts allowed."* ~
> *Unknown*

I may have tormented myself with beliefs like this. How am I supposed to do this?

With tapping, and mindfulness, I'm actually encouraged to allow the negative thoughts to come up. As I do this and tap, I actually honor all parts of me. Even the Debbie or Donny Downer part of me.

This part of me needs the most airtime initially, so I can stop tormenting myself with the belief that somehow, someway, I'm supposed to eradicate negative thoughts from my being. When I don't allow them their full expression, they stay stuck in my body and can cause all manner of ills.

Not allowing my truth, no matter how it sounds, just helps it to grow into a long-held resentment. This isn't good for anybody. It actually imprisons my emotions in my body and my being.

However, when I use tapping or mindfulness practices, I allow them all. With tapping I allow them and I tap while allowing them, and the amazing result is I begin to release my negative thoughts.

With mindfulness I allow them. I allow them to float by while noticing them. I can interrupt my negative thoughts with mental noting, where I just state the name of the emotion or state what's going on with one word. I might notice judging thoughts going by and I just stop and say, "Judging."

This simple practice creates a pattern interrupt while allowing what appears to be negative thought to surface. What a relief!

It's way too much unnecessary pressure to not allow negative thoughts. With tapping or the mental noting, I shift my negative thoughts by allowing them and interrupting them. This is so much easier.

THOUGHT FOR THE DAY*: I can't stop my thoughts, but I can interrupt them. This can make a big change within me the more I practice it.*

September 2

> *"It's okay to be a glow stick: Sometimes we have to break before we shine."* ~
> *Unknown*

Being human is an interesting prospect. Often how the desire for change seems to arise is out of desperation. When I feel desperate, I'm at a breaking point. Whatever has been going on is not working or is no longer working, and it's time to do something about it.

Often I get upset that I'm in this place where things aren't working for me, but what if this thing that's not working for me, this thing that seems to break me, is the very thing that brings me back to my true self?

What if the thing that's caused me the pain and the breaking, breaks me open to a deeper connection with a power greater than my human self?

What if the breaking open is the path to a greater understanding and new possibilities I just couldn't see before? In this way, the breaking open is orchestrated for my soul's evolution.

THOUGHT FOR THE DAY: *What if the very thing that has caused me to break is the very thing breaking me open to a deeper connection to a power greater than myself?*

September 3

"No one is you and that is your superpower." ~ Freepik

I might have a doppelganger running around the planet. Apparently, we all do. Unless I run into them, though, I'll never know for sure. Yet, even if I have a doppelganger, that person is not me. I will find people throughout my life I have a lot in common with. I might even find people who appear to be my twin from another mother in personality, but I'm still 100% uniquely me. Even identical twins have differences, you can see them and hear their personality differences when they talk.

So in all the world, there will never be another me, exactly as I am right now. If I take this in, it's actually amazing to ponder.

If I want to write a book, and there are thousands of books on the same topic, that need not stop me. If I'm not caught up in the world's view of competition, then I can realize that it doesn't matter how many other books there are out there on the same topic, there's still no one going to write the same book I will write. The book I write has my unique personality and spin on it, and it never needs to compete with anyone else's book.

This goes for anything I do. Only I can do it the way I do. That can take competition out of the equation. What if there are people out there waiting for what I have to share, even if it's just a smile on a train or an airplane? Even if they just see the smile in my eyes?

This is me, one of a kind.

THOUGHT FOR THE DAY: *What if today I can take a few moments and take in just how unique I really am?*

September 4

"Never regret being a good person to the wrong people." ~ Unknown

---

This is difficult, especially in the beginning. If someone treats me in a way that's hurtful for me, I should have my feelings.

It never works to tell myself that, despite how they treated me, I can be kind to them. If I try to force this on myself, I usually just clamp down on my true feelings and add to an already overloaded suppression load. If, however, I allow myself all of my feelings in a safe, healthy, and probably private way (with support, if needed), I get to feel all that I need to and as fully as possible. Tapping helps me move through this.

The beauty of allowing myself my truth in this way is I don't end up with stuck emotional energy within me.

I need not put a timeline on this. I need not tell myself I need to be over this by a certain date. I get to practice feeling my way through this until I sense that I'm complete.

A great way to know that I'm complete is I'll find that I'm not reactive with this same person. I feel free of any emotional ties that have bound me to them. They could even say something that I would have found hurtful in the past, and I either laugh about it or it just rolls off of me. This is true freedom. This is also very empowering me.

My process takes whatever it takes for me, and the more I honor myself in this way, the more emotional freedom I'll find. I can also know that sometimes the triggers with certain personalities are more volatile for me, and I seem to get triggered a lot faster with them. This is just letting me know there's a deeper wound here and it will require more tapping and releasing. It's also highly likely that the pricklier the personality for me, the more tapping and patience with myself it takes. It takes what it takes.

THOUGHT FOR THE DAY: *What if I find myself triggered and I remind myself to tap, even if it's after the fact? That is enough.*

September 5

"It's always the simple that produce the marvelous." ~ Amelia Barr

I might have the personality that can complicate a French fry. If that's the case, then I might not agree that the simple things produce the marvelous. It just hasn't been my experience.

What if I could experiment with this and just sit for one minute during a busy day and focus on my breath? Now I might feel like I could crawl out of my skin attempting this, or I might find that my mind is racing away on what I have to do next, but either way, I'm getting insight into my current state of internal affairs.

If I feel soothed, I might find I want to do more of these daily pauses. They do have the power to center and ground me, and who can't use more of that?

What if this is a simple experiment that can actually have a marvelous effect on me the more I practice it?

THOUGHT FOR THE DAY*: What if I can take the midday one-minute pause and just notice what happens within me?*

September 6

"Doubt kills more dreams than failure ever will." ~ Suzy Kassem

This is so true, and yet how do I stop myself from doubting? The quick answer is that I don't. What if I can remember this little ditty:

"I can't stop my thoughts, but I can interrupt them."

What a great reminder.

If I don't want to allow doubt to kill my dream, I might "try" to not doubt. This actually only makes the doubt stronger. It's the old saying, "Whatever you resist persists."

It is such a relief to know that I can't stop my thoughts of doubt, but I can interrupt them before they gain too much momentum. Initially, it's likely I will not catch the doubt that often. That doesn't matter because each time I do catch it and interrupt it, I see it more.

I need not pay attention to all my thoughts of doubt all day. That would drive me crazy. I just interrupt when I can, even if it's after the fact, because the more I do this, the easier it is to spot the doubt and the less it has a grip on me.

Mental noting is another great way to interrupt because it's even simpler than tapping, and I can do it in my head really easily. Here's how it works. When I catch myself doubting, I just say the word, "Doubting," either to myself or out loud—whichever works for me—and this powerfully interrupts the momentum of doubt.

Doubt might kill more dreams than failure ever will, but I can be ready to attend to my doubtful thoughts and ultimately not let doubt take me over.

THOUGHT FOR THE DAY: *What if I have moments of doubt today, I notice and I just say, "Doubting," and notice how it interrupts the flow of doubt.*

September 7

*"Your current situation is given to you
as an opportunity to re-evaluated what you
want." ~ Tashabee*

If I don't like what's happening in my life, tapping can help me to expose what is getting in my way. As I tap to relieve the stress and pressure I feel, this allows me access to the part of my brain that can re-evaluate and come up with solutions that work for me.

This is how all situations can become opportunities to re-evaluate. I get to see what I don't want in living color. The beauty of seeing what I don't want is it actually helps me to get closer to what I do want.

Over time, I make adjustments that help me move forward with a lot more ease.

THOUGHT FOR THE DAY: *What if seeing what I don't want is actually a steppingstone to seeing what I do want?*

September 8

"I'm still learning." ~ Michelangelo

What a great mantra. I could use this every day, all day long. It's true, too. I am always learning, and until I'm out of this body, I will be learning here in this form, in this lifetime.

Michelangelo was said to see the art within the marble. He would just remove the marble that would allow the sculpture to be seen. This is true of me in my emotional life.

Tapping and mindfulness both help me to remove the stagnant emotions blocking me from seeing my true self. As I clear out the learned limits, the true self comes through and life takes on a new quality. It can lead me to emotional intelligence and even a deepening of a connection with my soul.

Every experience I have gives me new opportunities to learn and evolve.

THOUGHT FOR THE DAY: *What if today is yet another day I will still be learning? I need not have all the answers.*

September 9

"You're not a mess. You're brave for trying." ~ Unknown

If someone would have told me this over and over again as I was growing up, it's likely I would be having a different life experience. Yet what if I came into this lifetime with a particular soul contract, meaning I came in with things I needed to experience for my soul's evolution? I came to learn to integrate new things.

The belief I (might) hold that I am a mess can feel true, but what if there's nothing wrong with having times where I feel like a mess? What if this is part of a recalibration process for my soul? What if I can remind the very human part of me that it is okay to feel like I'm a mess? This too shall pass, and I find I might not feel like a mess at all the next day.

This goes back to the idea that some days I feel more messy than others, and other days I feel grounded and not like a mess.

What if I can see that I am brave for experiencing my humanity and all that goes with this, including the emotions as part of my experience? What if I chose to be on this planet at this time because my soul knew that it was what I needed?

THOUGHT FOR THE DAY: *What if there's nothing wrong with the messy part of me? What if I am brave?*

September 10

"Never forget how wildly capable you
are." ~ Unknown

Within me, there is this wildly capable, all knowing, all seeing, wise part of me. It's my authentic self. I may have lost touch with this part of me, but it's always there. It's never gone, and it is always available to guide me. It's within me just waiting for me to tune back into it.

As I tune back into this part of me, I might ask for guidance. My impatience for an answer might kick in because the world's way is fast paced. It should be considered, though, that sometimes answers don't come because the timing isn't right yet. Things are lining up but, for the highest good to come into being, there's a wait period. These periods can be maddening when I first work with the guidance.

Learning to let go of my ego's agenda can feel like I'm doing something wrong. Sitting back and allowing what needs to come into my experience to come can be challenging. My ego mind rails and whines and tells me I'm being lazy and that I need to make it happen, and this language can feel right for a while. It feels right because it's what I'm used to, not because it means it's right.

To think that I can ask for guidance and the guidance doesn't always come right away is something to get used to. It's a new way of seeing things. The unhooking process is a challenging journey because the ego acts up and tell me what's what.

As I learn to recognize who is running my show, I unhook a little more. This allows things to fall into place.

THOUGHT FOR THE DAY*: What if trusting the guidance that comes is a process? As I learn to allow this force to lead me, things fall into place and my trust grows.*

September 11

"You're a fighter. Look at everything
you've overcome. Don't give up." ~ Olivia
Benson

Do I want to be a fighter? I would like to believe that I need not fight for things to work out for me. Isn't this a construct of the bully in my brain? It's always fighting with me. Do I have to overcome something to receive what's best for me? Isn't this a construct of the bully in my brain as well?

What if when I give up sometimes, that means I'm tired of the fight? What if giving up is my exhausted self's version of letting go? What if, as I'm throwing in the towel and waving the surrender flag, I become open to finding a better way? I can reach the place where I realize there's got to be a better way.

What if this is God, The Universe, my higher self, or whatever I called it, actually guiding me back home? It just uses exhaustion to get my attention because it works.

As I stop fighting and trying so hard, I find that my life unfolds in synchronistic ways.

THOUGHT FOR THE DAY: *What if today it's actually a good thing to give up because it means I am surrendering my way and my will to something so much greater?*

September 12

---

*"The happiness of your life depends on
the quality of your thoughts." ~ Pinterest*

Oh boy! No pressure there. So if I don't have good quality thoughts, my life won't be happy? What if I grew up not understanding how to feel happy or how to think well of myself or believe that there's a lot of good possible for me? Should I just hang my head and forget about it?

This idea that I have to have quality thoughts to be happy stresses me out. If my resting thought rate isn't so great, this would be very stressful for me. I might believe that I have to stop thoughts that aren't good. This can throw me into a spiritual bypass, where I deny negative thoughts and try to "just get happy."

The thing that's missed here is, once again, I can't actually stop my thoughts. It doesn't work. If I'm caught up in negative thoughts and think that I need to be more positive without attending to what's causing my negative thinking in the first place, I will further suppress the emotions tied to these thoughts.

If, however, I can take some of the pressure off myself and remind myself that I can't stop my negative thoughts, but I can interrupt, I can find immediate relief, which lowers the pressure I place on myself. To think that it's actually a good thing to go into my negative thoughts (i.e., my current truth) and use tapping to help me release them feels so much better than telling myself that my happiness depends on the quality of my thoughts. The irony is that as I go into my negative thoughts and release them, my resting thought rate becomes infinitely more positive over time without my "trying" to think positive or "trying" to deny the negative thoughts I have that are part of the human condition.

What a relief.

THOUGHT FOR THE DAY: *I can't stop my negative thoughts, but I can interrupt them with tapping and find relief.*

September 13

"I can and I will." ~ Gistping

Yikes! What if I find I can't so I won't? Is this okay? "I can and I will" sounds like the ego pounding its chest instead of being open to something that might be better for me and for my highest good. If I become fixated on how I think things should be, and I put much force and pressure to make it happen and it doesn't happen, how do I feel when "I can and will" turns into "I can't and I won't"? (Hint: I bet I feel bad.)

What if this is a great reminder that if something is not happening in the way I think it should and under my chosen timeline, it's actually not meant to? What if it's not meant to because of the spiritual concepts of Diving Timing (i.e., the synchronicity of the Universe) and Divine Order (i.e., the flow of the Spirit as we surrender to this guidance and direction). The timing isn't for the highest, and what I think I want is not in the flow for the highest.

I need not believe this, but what if I could just ponder whether it makes sense of not? Surrendering to a higher source (i.e., Divine Surrender) doesn't mean I do nothing. It means I act from inspiration rather than action that comes from me having to motivate myself to accomplish something, even though this something may not be in my best interest.

What if there really could be something better that will come when I get my agenda out of the way? It's just something to consider.

THOUGHT FOR THE DAY: *What if there really could be Divine Timing, Divine Order, and Divine Surrender?*

September 14

"Good Vibes Only "~ Unknown

Lord help me with this one. This is a spiritual bypass at its finest, and this is a big ask.

Good vibes only? How does one do this? Do they ever have bad vibe days? What do they do on their bad vibe days?

This doesn't consider the amazing palette of emotions I came installed with. Emotions all meant to be felt and felt fully. What if all of my emotions are what give me richness as a human?

If I attempt to have only good vibes, I actually cut-off a large part of me and make anything that appears to not be "good vibes" forbidden. Over time, these now "forbidden" emotions (bad vibes) need to go somewhere. This is where they leak out at very inopportune times.

So if I want to be a more well-rounded human, embracing both good and bad vibes and then attending to my bad vibes, so I don't wallow in them, is a good recipe for emotional fitness.

THOUGHT FOR THE DAY*: What if today I can embrace my good and not so good vibes and make them all okay?*

September 15

"Staying positive doesn't mean you have to be happy all the time. It means that even on hard days you know that there are better ones coming."
~ Unknown

This feels a lot better and a lot more doable. To think that every day has a variety of experiences—some which feel good, some that feel bad, and everything in between—feels real.

To have a hard day and to know that it won't last is a relief. This doesn't mean I have to like the hard days, or try to get happy about them, or even during a hard day try to see the good in it. It means that some days are easier and lighter and more enjoyable than others. It means that some days are harder and heavier and not as enjoyable as others. But both pass. That's the great news. Both pass and both come back around. That is the cycle of life.

As I learn to accept the cycles of life, I can find more balance and grounding, even when the hard days are at hand. They don't last. Acceptance softens everything.

THOUGHT FOR THE DAY: What if today I can remind myself that acceptance does soften everything?

September 16

> *"A negative mind will never give you a positive life."* ~ *pinterest.au*

Here we go again trying not to think negatively. I will keep this short and sweet.

There's nothing wrong with negative thinking, as long as I'm interrupting the patterns of negative thoughts so they don't stay stuck like glue and I wallow in them. As I allow whatever I'm feeling it's full expression, it does what it's meant to do—it moves on.

And I'm all the better for it.

THOUGHT FOR THE DAY: What if today I can do my best and just allow my feelings to move through me? I can use tapping if I need to assist myself in a fuller expression of them.

September 17

"Life isn't about waiting for the storm to pass. It's about learning to dance in the rain."

~ Vivian Greene

Finally, something that makes sense. Even if I can't dance in the rain just yet, I can learn to. As I learn to allow whatever is in my experience to just be what it is, and then allow myself to fully go into this experience, it moves on as it's intended to do.

Emotions don't get buried alive inside of me because I'm allowing them to be what they are and to be felt through to their completion. When I complete emotions, I move through them. They aren't buried alive inside of me. I become more emotionally intelligent and fit because I no longer have this epic buildup of emotions that have to get out somehow, some way.

I'm actually living more in the moment with my emotions and life experiences. This means I'm actually present for my life. Imagine that.

When I'm present for my life more often, I might find peace and contentment are in my experience. This can be a wonderful way to live. My life is richer.

THOUGHT FOR THE DAY*: What if my life becomes richer as I learn to dance with what's in front of me? I'm dancing in any weather pattern.*

September 18

"Don't be impressed by: Money,
Followers, Degrees, Titles. Be impressed by:
Kindness, Integrity, Humility, Generosity."
~ Unknown

Being impressed with these things is following the ego's desires. The ego is a drug pusher. It pushes me to get more degrees, to add letters behind my name so I have more credibility, to work harder, to make more money. If I keep following this agenda, I can end up exhausted and thinking there's got to be more to life than this.

It's often out of this exhaustion I let go. I don't try to let go; I just do. I surrender in a way because I just can't keep going on in this way. It feels too empty, and the truth is there are never enough titles, degrees, or money to quench the ego's desires. They are endless.

If, however, in my surrendering I open up, guidance comes to me. I might overhear something on the radio, or hear someone talking to someone else, or see a billboard, or see something on TV, and in an instant, I know this is something I can take a step towards. I may not know where it leads, but I find I have this urge to do it anyway and just see what happens.

This isn't the way of the ego; this is the way of spirit. The more I try this, the better I find I feel, and my life blossoms in ways far better than my ego driven desires can take me.

THOUGHT FOR THE DAY: *What if today I can check in on whether I'm pushing the ego's desires or following the promptings of my spirit?*

September 19

"Until you make the unconscious conscious, it will direct your life and you will call it fate." ~ C.G. Jung

---

This is one benefit of tapping. While tapping, I can have the experience of unconscious thoughts surfacing. Memories I have forgotten about can come up because they are linked to whatever emotional experience I am attending to in the moment.

Tapping allows the unconscious to become conscious, which is where I can attend to it and release it so it doesn't run me, and I end up considering well-rehearsed thought patterns my fate.

I get to allow whatever needs to come up to come up. This allows whatever comes up to move on and be released. To use tapping as a safety net that actually goes into my unconscious and reveals what I need to see to find relief is actually kind of amazing.

This simple technique of tapping on meridian points while expressing my truth allows my brain to uproot my unconscious programming so I can be released from the limits it's placed on my life. This opens me up to a fuller, richer life experience. I'll have that please.

THOUGHT FOR THE DAY*: What if I could trust that whatever surfaces with tapping is what needs to surface to help set me free?*

September 20

"I'm starting over. A new pattern of thoughts. A new wave of emotions. A new connection to the world. A new belief system in myself." ~ Overlyxclusive

---

This mentality indicates that I am following the guidance of my soul. It's like the ultimate do-over.

Maybe I reached the point where I just felt empty inside and realized there has to be more. Maybe what I'm doing has not been working for me, and I'm tired of trying too hard and working so hard and not seeing the good come from all of that work.

What if when things don't work out the way I learned to believe they should, this happens not because I'm doing anything wrong, but because I'm meant to follow a new way, with new thought patterns and a deeper connection to my emotions and my inner world? All with less connection to the world's agenda for me?

This can be the gateway to a freer, fuller, more fulfilling life experience as I learn to follow the signs that come.

THOUGHT FOR THE DAY: *What if today I can pay attention and notice the signs?*

September 21

"We must be willing to let go of the life
we planned so as to have the life that is
waiting for us." ~ Joseph Campbell

This can throw me into a tailspin upon first visiting this concept. In a world that teaches me that what will be is up to me, letting go can fill me with fear. My head may spin with tales of woe over not getting the things I believe that I want in my life. What often gets missed in this do-it-yourself world I live in is that there is a force of good that knows what's best, and it has a plan that can unfold for me. A plan beyond my wildest dreams from a limited human perspective, yet I grasp so hard for what I think is best I can't even see it could be possible there is something so much greater, so much more suited for me, if I could only release the death grip on how I think things should be.

Letting go is a process. The very human side of me needs to be honored for all its fears and concerns so I can release them and open up to the life this force of good has lined up for me. I'm not taught to live in this way in the world of pushing the ego's want list.

As I learn to let go of the want list, I see and feel there is so much more that can come in because I open to it. The beauty is all I need to start with is the willingness. The rest will line up and be shown in the right time in the right way. Until that happens, I have tapping to help quell my doubts and fears so I can continue to open up to what wants to come into my experience.

THOUGHT FOR THE DAY*: What if there is a force for good that has my back, knows what's best, and is waiting to show me the way to what's best for me? I need not believe this yet, but what if I can open just a little to this possibility?*

September 22

"Do what you can, where you are, with what you have." ~ Theodore Roosevelt

---

Teddy Roosevelt might be talking about an aspect of acceptance. If I follow this advice and do what I can, where I can, with what I have, I might be making the best of things in the moment.

Instead of railing against what I can't do, what I don't have, and wherever I might find myself, I go with what is. It speaks to a level of acceptance of "what is" that can create a sense of peace for me.

But I am always allowed my truth with tapping. Tapping is this safety net that allows me to go deeper into my emotions, through any experience or circumstance, and release what I need to rather than continue to bury whatever feelings surface. I always get my truth with tapping. By honoring my truth and giving it a voice, I create more calmness within me. I become less reactive and more responsive to whatever is happening in life.

In this way, I am more likely to accept what is in the moment. It doesn't mean I have to resign myself to what is and never hold space for things to change or become better. Quite the contrary. As I keep giving myself my truth, I find that I'm capable of doing what I can when I get the impulse to take inspired action. I find that where I am is the place I'm meant to be for now.

The more I give myself the gift of acceptance, the more emotionally free and balanced I become. Thank you, Teddy.

THOUGHT FOR THE DAY: *What if I ask for acceptance for what is, for now?*

September 23

"Be patient. Everything is coming together." ~ Unknown

I might be a professional doubter that good things are happening for me, especially if I've lived a life where this doesn't feel like it's the case. I may see others living lives that appear to be good, but this good ship seems to pass me by.

What if all the beliefs that I've been living under can be drilled down to well-practiced thought patterns I learned a long time ago? These thought patterns became adopted by my unconscious and are now my current programmed set of beliefs, but they aren't more than well-rehearsed thought patterns.

Beliefs are just thoughts that I've been thinking over and over again.

I can use tapping to help me to interrupt these thought patterns, and the more I do this, the less true these thoughts feel. The less true they feel, the more evidence I have that my physiology is changing. This means these beliefs are being uprooted so that there's space to experience something different. Something better.

This can help me to be more patient, and it can help me to be more open to everything really being lined up and coming together for my highest good.

THOUGHT FOR THE DAY: *What if today I can interrupt repetitive thoughts that don't serve me?*

September 24

"Darkness cannot drive out darkness: only light can do that. Hate cannot drive out hate: only love can do that." ~ Martin Luther King, Jr.

Martin Luther King Jr. spoke such words of truth. If I remain locked in the darkness, all I get is more darkness. If, however, I use tapping and go into the darkness to come through the darkness through the releasing of the dark thoughts that can plaque my psyche, these thoughts find their way out of my mind and thus are released.

As I release more of the darkness within me, I need not try to bring lightness into my being because the light is always there and already within me. What happens is now that the darkness is diminished, my natural positive lightness of being has the space to shine and come through me.

This differs greatly from trying to think positive. This is hacking away at the darkness that's been instilled in me by going into the darkness within me so it can be released. I have nothing to fear about the darkness, especially as I go into it intentionally and consciously so it can be released.

THOUGHT FOR THE DAY: *What if the way out of the darkness is through it, so it can be uprooted and released?*

September 25

> *"I have a happy personality with a heavy soul. Sometimes, it gets weird."*
>
> *~ Gauri Shanker Singh*

What if there is no such thing as a heavy soul? What if the dark night of the soul is misinterpreted? What if there is no dark night of the soul because the soul doesn't have darkness? What if it's the bully in my brain (the ego) that carries heaviness and darkness?

As I become mindful of when the bully is having one of its many episodes, I can recognize it for what it is: an aspect of the ego filling me with fear.

As I catch it in the act, I allow my healthy adult self to take over so the emotional intelligent part of me takes the lead in my life once again. The more this happens, the more I find that the force of good speaks through synchronicities.

THOUGHT FOR THE DAY*: What if the darkness is always from the ego, and as I catch it in the act of the fear mongering it likes to dish out, I see a better way?*

September 26

"A winner is a dreamer who never gives up." ~ Nelson Mandela

Dang, we're back to the winners and losers thing. I might love Nelson Mandela and his incredible story, but I don't want to keep thinking in terms of winners and losers anymore. This sets me up for competition, and when competition reigns, there is no space for cooperation. I want to live from a place of cooperation rather than the defeating world of winners and losers. Otherwise, someone's always got to be on top, and then someone always has to be behind.

I want to learn to lift myself up and cooperate with myself instead of competing with anyone, not even myself. The world of winners and losers is a world the bully thrives in. I don't want the bully in my brain to thrive anymore. It's had center stage for far too long now.

What if I can be a dreamer who allows something greater than myself to lead me? If I'm meant to move on to something better, then I let go of what's not working so I can embrace what is for my highest and best good.

THOUGHT FOR THE DAY*: I release the world of winners and losers and seek the world where cooperation is queen.*

September 27

"Karma. What goes around comes around. Keep your circle positive. Speak good words. Think good thoughts. Do good deeds." ~ powerofpositivity.com

---

No pressure here. What do I do on the days and nights I can't seem to eke out a positive thought? This is where tapping can be my best ally. It allows me, once again, to go into the negative thoughts I have and own them so they can be released.

Tapping doesn't ask me to just think positive, happy thoughts. Tapping asks me to go into what is disturbing and disrupting me, so I can be free of the grip my unattended truth can have on me.

I'm allowed every thought and every feeling without exception, and in doing so I find peace and emotional freedom on the other side of the negative. The way out is through, and with tapping I go through the fire and out to the other side where the force of good can give.

THOUGHT FOR THE DAY*: What if what is gone through is released? Especially with eyes wide open to the experience.*

September 28

"Freedom requires that you discover your own inner language - your own life rules - your own vision." ~ Zephyr Bloch Jorgensen

This is a key to a more fulfilling life experience. As I continue to release the learned limits I adopted, my unique inner language and vision come bubbling up from within. This can be aided as I learn to listen to the force for good who speaks to and comes through me. Life takes on new meaning as I continue to unhook from the world's view of how life should work for me.

I no longer want to adopt the programming from a world that doesn't listen to the inner voice—the force for good. The world is constantly pushing the ego's plan often devoid of what matters.

Breaking free from the world's view is its own journey because the majority of people listen to and adopt views about life that leave many of us worn out from all the trying to make things happen and the trying to manifest the ego's desires. It sets us up on a treadmill of pushing.

As I learn to listen to my inner wisdom that comes through me from the force of good, I see things in a new way. Overtime I see the programming that the world pushes, and I reach a place where I do discover the inner language and vision that flows through me for my highest good. It may feel challenging at first because of all the learned limits, but I have tapping to help me move through them so I can hear my inner wisdom more and more.

THOUGHT FOR THE DAY: *What if I can just notice the voice of the world I live in? Notice the pushing energy, notice the shoulds, the shouldn't. Just pay attention.*

September 29

> *"Never doubt what one prayer can do."*
> *~ @TrustGodbro*

Oh, I may doubt the power of prayer, and if I have, I've made myself wrong for this. This is the first place to start.

Any exacting statements like "never doubt the power of prayer" can be a set-up for major disappointment. I can feel bad about myself because I may doubt the power of prayer.

This is why tapping can be so liberating. I get to speak my unadulterated, unedited truth, so I can be free of the hold it has on me when I hold it in and try to act like I shouldn't doubt. I may have been taught that the God of my understanding never wants me to doubt. If so for me, what if I can consider this belief that God, or whatever I chose to call it, who wants me to never doubt is man-made by an ego-based culture? I may have learned this consideration is blasphemous, but once again, if God or this force for good has a lot of rules and commandments I need to follow to be acceptable, it might be time to rethink it.

It's likely I'll have to work through my programming around this, so I soften my self-blame because I'm not a full-on believer. Talk about competition. I'm a believer (winner), you're not (loser). This becomes an exclusive club that God has set-up.

I really might want to ponder that the force for good that created so much beauty in the world has a member's only VIP club that people get excluded from if they're deemed as not being on their best behavior. This might trip my triggers, but I can tap to find soothing for this and see what comes up for me.

I would prefer to believe in a force of love all-inclusive rather than a crazy force that dubs winners and losers based on some merit system.

THOUGHT FOR THE DAY: *What if there is a force of good that is all-inclusive?*

September 30

"The two things in life you are in
control over are your attitude and your
effort." ~ Billy Cox

This may not feel true for me. If I'm honest with myself, I would have to say that I'm not in control of my emotions. More often than not, it's the other way around; my emotions run me. Especially when I'm triggered. If this is true for me, it's only because I haven't been shown how to attend to my emotional landscape, so it allows me to put my healthy self back in the driver's seat.

As for the effort part, I hear a lot of talk from the world about how hard work pays off. The thing is I know many people, maybe myself included, who have worked hard their whole lives and still don't feel like they're successful or living a good life.

How could there be time for a good life if someone is working hard a lot? What if there's a big difference between working hard and working from inspiration? If I'm caught up in the hard work belief system, then there are plenty of times I have to "motivate" myself to do something. This can be tiring and painful. What if hard work isn't optimal? What if there's another way to see this? What if, as I act from inspired thoughts, things are a lot easier? I'm invigorated, and hard work isn't necessary. These aren't ideas I've heard thrown around in this world often. To sit quietly and connect with my inner wisdom and then wait for right actions to be shown can feel counterintuitive, though it's actually not. It might take me some time to trust this, but that's okay too. I can take all the time I need to unhook from a world that's wired backwards. I like the idea that I can learn to believe that there's a big difference between hard work and inspired action.

THOUGHT FOR THE DAY*: What if today I can entertain the idea that inspired actions comes directly from a force for good?*

October

October 1

> *"Our ego is our silent partner...too often with a controlling interest."* ~ *Cullen Hightower*

This silent partner is like a nightmare of a boss. It's loud and obnoxious and a colossal pain in the ass. It wants to be in charge all the time, and it always thinks it knows best, all while feeding me the absolute worst possible scenarios.

It can be loud and in my face and takes on this bully characteristic, or it can be subtler, sneakier, rational sounding and very evidence based. It will bully me into submission, or it will use evidence to show me how I'm messing up all the time. This ego is not my friend. It does the opposite of the force of good. It shows me why everything is impossible and what things will not work out.

Depending on how my ego comes to me—in bully mode or evidence-based, rational mode—I know it's operating in my psyche by how I feel. If I'm feeling bad about myself, the ego is in charge. That's why the more I witness who is running my show and interrupt it and take back the reins, the less active the ego can be in my life day to day.

It won't ever go away, but it can be managed so that I'm not so affected by it. This is more than good enough. The more I catch it and interrupt it, the less weight it carries in my life and the better I feel.

THOUGHT FOR THE DAY*: What if today when I catch the ego taking over, I can pause and tell it to take a back seat? It may sneak back in again and again, but that's okay. Catching it is a great practice.*

October 2

---

*"The ego wants quantity, but the soul
wants quality." ~ Unknown*

This is very true. The ego (the bully) is never content, never satisfied. As soon as one thing is accomplished it says, "What's next?" There's never enough of anything for my ego. It preaches, "Never enough," all the time.

It points out all that's missing in my life and in me. It literally beats me up and then comes back and kicks me when I'm down. It can sound demonic or pull the evidence-based torment over and over and over.

When it sounds demonic, it sounds like, "You'll never make it. Who do you think you are? You're a loser." It's in my face filling me with negativity.

When it sounds reasonable, it sounds like, "You should really call your mother. You shouldn't let them get to you. You know that didn't work out last time." It gives me evidence and sounds reasonable, but I still feel bad.

It thinks it's huge, but it's just loud. It's a cranky, punitive voice that feeds me the shit show.

When I'm feeling exhausted and yet I'm still pushing myself to do more, this is the ego. I want to learn to allow my soul to take over and be the voice I hear more and more. A great way to help this to happen is to keep catching the ego in the act and tapping to find relief. The more I do this, the less active it is, and the more I can hear my soul speaking through me. My soul speaks of ease, of acceptance, of patience, of worthiness, and of deserving of all that is good. This voice can become the predominant voice I pay attention to just by tapping through the darkness the ego feeds me.

THOUGHT FOR THE DAY: *What if I can remind myself that I need not be positive? Just interrupting the negative self-talk of the ego is enough to allow my soul to be heard.*

October 3

"Our ego is the part of us that cares about our status and what people think."

Brene Brown

Anytime I care too much about how I look, the car I drive, the home I live in, the work I do, and what other people think, my ego (the bully) is in charge. It's great to see this because being aware is the most important part of this process. It doesn't mean that things will change for me right away. I can be guaranteed that they won't change right away. But if I keep noticing and I keep making little shifts with tapping, a day will come when I notice that the bully is not in charge as much. I'll notice that, when it's feeding me the shit show, I just don't believe it as deeply. This is evidence I'm changing my physiology and thus changing my thoughts.

The more I keep noticing and tapping, the less and less strong the bully is in my life and the more I feel lighter and freer. This is a path to a much better way of living.

THOUGHT FOR THE DAY*: What if today it's enough to know what the bully is feeding me, without trying to change a thing? I just tap to help it find its release.*

October 4

> *"The ego says, "Once everything falls into place, I'll feel peace." Spirits says, "Find your peace and then everything will fall into place." ~ Marianne Williamson*

This can be a moment of awakening. My ego is often telling me to fix myself enough so I can manifest the things I want. It will tell me if I just align my thoughts better, if I visualize what I want more often, what I want will come.

But often this isn't the case. I can try to manifest and visualize until my eyes go cross-eyed, or work hard to keep a high vibration, and I'm still not getting what I want.

If, on the other hand, I want to feel peace more than acquire anything on my list of wants, the weird thing is that my list of wants seems to come to me in an even better way. I've genuinely let go, and I've released attachment to a particular outcome. I've released pushing the ego's agenda. If something still doesn't come, it's not meant to. It's not for my highest good.

As I find more peace, then everything does fall into place.

THOUGHT FOR THE DAY*: What if today I can ask for assistance from the force of good to help me let go and allow in what is for my highest?*

October 5

"Life is not accomplishing some special work but attaining to a degree of consciousness and inner freedom which is beyond all works and attainments." ~
Thomas Merton

I would like to choose inner freedom and peace over anything from the material world. Inner freedom brings with it detachment and a detached mind is free.

The world often tells me I need to focus on what I want and never waver, and only then will it come. After a while this sounds tiring and it sounds this way because it is. It's letting me know the ego is pushing its agenda in my life and that always feels unfulfilling.

I may not understand how to detach, but I can always ask for guidance and watch what guidance comes. In this way, I learn to detach because I'm shown the way, and as I learn how to detach from specific outcomes in my life, there is space for new possibilities to come into being.

THOUGHT FOR THE DAY*: What if today I can just notice when I'm attached to a particular outcome and just let that be enough?*

October 6

"Sometimes you have to let go to be free." ~ Unknown

How do I let go?

What if these steps can help me learn to let go?

1) *Even if I don't feel this yet, what if I can write down what I'm attached to and then rip it up in an act of letting it go to a higher being?*
2) *What if I can ask for assistance in helping me to believe I can trust in the process of turning it over to a higher being?*
3) *What if I can tap when I feel doubt or fear surfacing?*

What if I can wash, rinse, and repeat these steps as often as I need to?

THOUGHT FOR THE DAY*: What if I can try this once today?*

October 7

"The ego wants me to think I'm in constant danger." ~ Pam Grout

---

I might know this from how much constant, low-grade fear I live with. While it might not be full-blown fear that demands attention, the low-grade fear of the ego shows up in the incessant mind chatter that can plague me daily. It sounds like:

"You can't do that."

"That's not going to work out."

"Are you sure you want to do that?"

"Oh, that's not smart."

"What were you thinking?"

These are examples of the subtle, sneaky ways these thoughts can keep fear alive in me.

What makes it tricky is this incessant chatter often goes unnoticed. I might not feel well emotionally, or I might not feel very hopeful for the future, but I don't see this because the thoughts just keep coming and I can become so used to them that I'm not conscious of what's being fed to my psyche.

As I wake up to this incessant chatter that induces fear daily, I can go through a period where I'm overwhelmed with how incessant it is. I am bringing the unconscious out into the open, and this is where I can change things. As I pay attention to my thoughts, I have the advantage of tapping through them so I can send them on their way, and they aren't the predominant thoughts anymore. This allows fear to lose its grip on me, and I notice I'm feeling better and more hopeful. It's so worth attending to, so I can live more fully.

THOUGHT FOR THE DAY: *What if today I can just notice my thoughts?*

October 8

"The cave you fear to enter holds the treasure you seek."

~ Joseph Campbell

Is this another way to tell me that if something is outside of my comfort zone, I need to do it anyway? A great first step, if this is the case, is to tap through my fears around the situation I'm shying away from.

As I tap, I attend to the fear, and the fear finds its way through me. Just as it's meant to do. As the fear loses its grip on me, and it's intensity becomes less overwhelming, my nervous system soothes, my cortisol (the stress hormone) level drops, and I have access to the part of my brain that can come up with creative, far less stressful solutions.

In this way, I don't have to "go outside my comfort zone" to act because I'm creating a more comfortable environment for myself before I have to act. I might not be free of fear, but I can feel fear and still act. I can use tapping anytime I need to, to help me to soften my fears of anything.

Tapping has a cumulative effect, so I can start more actions in my life with a lot less fear ruling me. I could enter many caves if I chose to and find the treasure I am seeking, and maybe the most important treasure is less fear.

THOUGHT FOR THE DAY*: What if tapping can be my greatest help when fear is present?*

October 9

"Find a place inside where there's joy, and the joy will burn out the pain."

~ Joseph Campbell

I love this, and yet I want to know how to find this place of joy inside of me. Especially if I've lived a life that's been anything but joyful.

Mediation, mindfulness, mindfulness meditation, and tapping are just some tools I can use to reconnect with my authentic self and the joy that actually abounds within me.

Tapping is a great tool to attend to the very human part of me that gets caught up in the world. Tapping allows me to quiet the bully in my brain and soothe my wounded inner child.

As I attend to these parts of me, I find relief and release. As I find these, what happens is, without even really "trying," I feel more moments of genuine joy, peace, contentment, and fulfillment. All qualities that can get lost in a world that promotes competition and getting mine. I see that, no matter what the world teaches, in my world things can be far more uplifting and fulfilling, and even joyful.

This doesn't mean, however, that I should believe that I always need to live in a state of joy. I'm still in this human experience and all that goes with that, so as I continue to allow myself my truth, I learn to be far more accepting of myself, and this leads to genuine self-love. And that's something that opens me up to more joy.

THOUGHT FOR THE DAY: *As I learn to accept myself as I am, I learn to love myself, and this allows me to access the joy inside.*

October 10

'It isn't what you have or who you are
or where you are or what you are doing that

makes you happy or unhappy. It is what you
think about it.' ~ Dale Carnegie

When I listen to the bully in my brain, it doesn't matter how much of anything I have, I'm never fulfilled. I'm always in the race to the next attainment to quell the bully's incessant chatter.

This is why I hear about people who appear to have it all and yet they are miserable. They are in pursuit of things that the world of the ego teaches, and though it might be temporarily fulfilling, it can't last. It can't last because of what Catherine Ponder once stated, "Whatever the ego creates, the ego can lose."

Fear of loss comes into play, and this leaves them feeling anxious and afraid of loss. This is the world of lack. It's the way the world thinks about it, and thus the way I learn to think about myself and my place in this world.

It's no one's fault. It's impossible to be in this world and not become a product of this environment. This is why it's so important for me to pay attention to who's running my show, the bully, or the wounded child. Once I know who's in charge, I use tapping to find relief. This allows me to move through the limitations I've learned that hold me captive.

As I honor my own journey and my process, life opens up for me in new ways, and my trust in a better way gets established.

THOUGHT FOR THE DAY: *It's not about status. It's not about anything the ego pushes on me. It's about how I think about it all that creates hell or heaven on earth for me. Tapping helps me to see and thus think in new ways so much better for me.*

October 11

"I tried to contain myself... but I escaped!"

~ Gary Paulsen

Being appropriate comes to mind when I hear this quote. I live in a world that preaches "being appropriate" to the point of losing myself. I often pay the price because of this idea that being appropriate is best. Yet this can actually inhibit me from honoring my truth. My unadulterated truth.

The world can be so exacting in its preaching about being nice, being kind, and being the first to forgive, and though these things are well meaning, it can inhibit me from feeling fully. Feeling fully is a way to get in touch with myself, and a means to escape society's preaching that have me putting a lid on my truth.

The saying, "The truth will set you free," applies for my healing journey. Tapping allows my truth so it is incredibly healing for me. This also allows me to learn to speak my truth in an emotional healthy way the more I release the truths stored in my body.

I escape societal convention for my truth. I learn to live true to myself and set myself free with no need to contain myself anymore. I see the effects that containing my truth has done and now I want to live my truth and honor myself.

THOUGHT FOR THE DAY: *My truth will set me free. I can use tapping to help me give myself my truth.*

October 12

---

*"The Universe has shaken you to
awaken you, and it's not punishment it's a
lesson."*

~ Mastin Kipp

As a human on this planet, I am subject to this human experience and all that goes along with that. Emotions, challenges, excitement, hope, doubt, lack of trust, trust, and so much more.

What if my soul came into this lifetime to evolve? What if what helps my soul evolve is life experiences that can both uplift me and challenge me? What if this is how I evolve as a human and as a soul? If I believe things happen to me because I'm being punished or because I'm just not getting it right, then I suffer. If whatever is coming into my experience has been chosen on a soul level, I'm less likely to condemn and judge myself. When challenges happen, something deeper is happening for me, on a soul level.

Life as a human is riddled with judgement, competition, and being hard on myself, just to name a few, yet as I practice acceptance about what I experience, I see that things are awakening me rather than from any punishment. This creates more ease and less stress.

THOUGHT FOR THE DAY: *What if the Universe is helping me to awaken by my soul's request?*

October 13

> *"When we are ready to make positive change in our lives, we attract whatever we need to help us." ~ Louise Hay*

When I want to change my life, I may not realize it, but I'm actually setting an intention. Without knowing it, I am asking for help. I've decided that things need to change, and it's unlikely that I know where to begin. I just know things need to change.

This decision creates an opening for me to receive guidance. Suddenly, I find a step that gets revealed. I might overhear a conversation. I might see a billboard with just the needed words. I might see a bumper sticker or see an ad for exactly what I need, or I might hear something that helps me.

Things seem to drop in my lap. The guidance just comes. Instead of pushing, things fall into place. What if this is the way it's always been intended to be?

THOUGHT FOR THE DAY: *What if my life unfolds with grace and ease?*

October 14

"The Universe is on your side so ask for guidance."

~ Tao of Dana

What a great follow up from yesterday's message. Now, I may not believe this yet, but what if it could be possible that the Universe is on my side and has my back and guides my way as I open to it?

Einstein once said, "The most important decision we make is whether we believe we live in a friendly or hostile universe."

My answer to this tells me my core belief. If I believe the Universe is friendly, then I believe I can ask for guidance. If I believe the Universe is hostile, then I will witness hostile, fearful things in my life. I won't trust that help is available, and I must use my force of will to "create" what I want. Even then it still may not happen.

If I can entertain the idea that the Universe is friendly and it does guide me, then my life can feel so much lighter and freer in every way. And, like yesterday's message, what if this is the way things are meant to be? I need not believe this yet, but I like that this could be possible.

THOUGHT FOR THE DAY: *What if the Universe is friendly and really can guide my way?*

October 15

"New Beginnings are often disguised as painful endings.

~ Lao Tzu

When things aren't working out for me, I can go down the rabbit hole of despair and pain, and I have a right to my feelings.

Tapping is a highly effective tool that helps me to allow my despair and pain so I can move beyond it. This allows me to see things from a fresh perspective. I see with new eyes. I've cleared the cobwebs of emotions and honored myself by doing so, and now I can find the blessing that comes in the disguise of an ending.

What if the reason something didn't work out, or the reason there was an ending, was because there is something even better lining up for me? As I see this as a possibility, I'm open to receiving the blessings.

Over time, I trust that if things aren't working out, it's because they're not meant to. They're not meant to because I need to make room for what is to come. I like this idea a lot. It sure feels better than the idea that endings are just painful, period. There's really so much more going on.

THOUGHT FOR THE DAY: *What if what appears to be a problem is just a blessing in disguise?*

October 16

"When you hold resentment toward another, you are bound to that person or condition by an emotional link that is stronger than steel. Forgiveness is the only way to dissolve that link and get free."

~ Catherine Ponder

The New Thought Movement, Law of Attraction, and religion talk about the importance of forgiveness. Just like this quote suggests. The challenge is, if I haven't allowed myself the fullness of my emotions when I feel hurt or betrayed by someone, forgiveness can feel as far from me as the stars.

Sometimes my attachment to non-forgiveness is the only way I feel some sense of power over what has happened. If I try to force myself to forgive before I've allowed myself my truth and my emotional experience, it doesn't work. It's not genuine. It's like forgiving someone while my teeth are gritted and I'm seething with resentment. If I will forgive someone, I want the freedom that comes with this for myself. I want to know that I have forgiven them with ease. I want to know that my forgiveness comes because I've honored myself fully and thus freed myself of the emotions that tie me to non-forgiveness.

As I give myself my full emotional experience, I actually complete my emotional experience which allows forgiveness to come with no forcing or trying. This is true emotional freedom.

THOUGHT FOR THE DAY: *I allow in forgiveness by honoring myself and my emotions fully.*

October 17

> *"I detach myself from preconceived outcomes and trust that all is well. Being myself allows the wholeness of my unique magnificence to draw me in those directions most beneficial to me and to all others. This is really the only thing I have to do. And within that framework, everything that is truly mine comes into my life effortlessly, in the most magical and unexpected ways imaginable, demonstrating every day the power and love of who I truly am.*
>
> *~ Anita Moorjani*

This is so beautiful and is something I aspire to achieve. It's important to know that detaching is its own journey. It's not like I can just detach from something I've been attached to. Learning to let go of preconceived outcomes is another part of the journey to detaching.

I may have a lot of momentum going that keeps me attached to outcomes. Tapping can help me to unhook from being attached. As I own my attachments, and tap through them, they lift on their own. I find evidence this is happening as I notice that I'm becoming less attached to particular outcomes and more open to receiving guidance as to what needs to come.

I honor myself and thus know myself and live true to myself.

This brings with it the effortlessness that Anita Moorjani talks about, where things work out for me in ways that amaze me. I follow the intuitive impulses that come and act when I feel inspired to, and magic seems to happen as things do unfold in ways that seemed unimaginable.

THOUGHT FOR THE DAY*: As I continue to awaken to the truth of my being, I realize this is the way it's always been meant to be.*

October 18

"Why are you trying so hard to fit in when you were born to stand out?"

~ Ian Wallace, What a Girl Wants

Could this be true?

In a world that teaches me to fit in, this can feel counterintuitive. But what if there is a fraction of truth in what is being said here? What if my journey is unique? It may look like anyone else's, but what if it's never been intended to be like anyone else's? What if there is a way that's meant just for me? What if I find I step on a very different path?

Maybe it's a path that's very different from what my parents, my family, or society has wanted for me. What if it can feel very unsettling at first, only because it doesn't fit into what the culture teaches me? What if, over time, it feels so much clearer and just right for me?

I like that my path is unique, and it need never look like anyone else's, ever.

THOUGHT FOR THE DAY: *What if today I can consider the thought that my path need never look like anyone else's?*

October 19

> *"I can't say this strongly enough, but our feelings about ourselves are actually the most important barometer for determining the condition of our lives."*
>
> *~ Anita Moorjani*

If I've lived on this planet any length of time, it's highly likely that I've adopted wrong thinking about myself. I've learned to believe that I'm limited, that I need to look a certain way, have a particular career, and have a certain status to be of value. As if my value has anything to do with these things or things like this.

So this wrong thinking I've learned to believe about myself needs to be shifted. Tapping provides me with a powerful tool to release this wrong thinking so the truth of myself has the space to come up from within me. I need not try to increase my self-esteem or self-confidence. As the wrong thinking gets cleared out of the way, I feel confident without trying to be confident. ⟦SEP⟧In this way, my feelings about myself improve dramatically, and this helps all areas of my life to improve.

THOUGHT FOR THE DAY: *What if I can tap when I notice I'm not feeling good about myself and know this is all I need to do right now?*

October 20

"The word "receive" means "to accept."

~ Catherine Ponder

I might struggle with allowing myself to receive, and if I am, it makes sense. The world often pitches a lifestyle and a way of being that carries no resonance with me. I might tell myself there's something wrong with me because I can't seem to create the life the world tells me I should want and have.

If I'm bumping up against this, my ability to receive is limited.

But if I can learn to accept myself in any moment, exactly as I am, this allows me to receive more goodness into my world. As I learn to accept more, I open myself to receive more.

This might not be what Catherine Ponder intended, but this is a perfect example of me learning to accept myself and that I may see something differently from someone else. This is absolutely as it should be.

As I learn to accept myself more, I open to receive more. I like this idea a lot. And learning to accept myself more is a journey of accepting what is, exactly as it is, in any moment. It's a practice I can do every day.

THOUGHT FOR THE DAY*: What if I open myself to receiving more through accepting myself more every day?*

October 21

"I believe that the greatest truths of the universe don't lie outside, in the study of the stars and the planets. They lie deep within us, in the magnificence of our heart, mind, and soul. Until we understand what is within, we can't understand what is without."

~ Anita Moorjani

This is what tapping can bring me to; the ability to see life and my place in it from a different perspective. As I use tapping to free myself from the learned limits I got programmed to take on, I not only become more emotionally intelligent and emotionally fit, but I might find I open up to a greater sense of truth that can only come from within me.

This greater sense of truth is always within me. It always has been, and it always will be.

I lost access to this inner knower over time, due to the congestion of limiting beliefs from a culture that values the outer, material world. Beliefs about what's appropriate or socially acceptable. Beliefs about gender, race, sexuality, health, and what a successful life should include.

As I tap through my learned limits, I open to my authentic self. I see that life need not be as hard as I was taught it is. Things lighten up for me and overtime and I see this is the way life is meant to be. I'll notice that my life unfolds with more ease. I notice that I'm feeling fulfillment from the simpler things because I'm connecting to my soul.

THOUGHT FOR THE DAY: *What if tapping helps me to reconnect with the magnificence of my heart, mind, and soul?*

October 22

"*All the gods, all the heavens, all the hells, are within you.*"

~ *Joseph Campbell*

Many of the world's religions teach about heaven and hell as actually physical places. God's personality is very human. God is a male. God chooses sides in a war. God yield's power over those who displease Him. Those who do please Him better keep one eye open because at any point God can ensue His wrath on the person of His choice. There are rules that must be followed to maintain my worthy status, and I better pay homage to Him in the proper way with the proper words, or else.

Another option is Law of Attraction. This Law is very similar to the God of many religions because if my life isn't turning out the way I want it to, then that falls solely on my shoulders. It's my fault because I'm not aligning correctly or visualizing enough.

What Joseph Campbell is talking about is that my life here can be heaven on earth or hell on earth depending on how I'm seeing it at any moment. If I don't get what I want, and I blame myself for this, this is hell on earth. If I don't get what I want and I tell myself that I'm not getting it because the god of my understanding is lining something so much better up for me, then my life feels more like heaven on earth.

The god of my understanding is likely what I learned about God as I was growing up. I get to go within and feel what God is like for me as I open to this. God might be something mind-blowingly different than I was raised to believe.

THOUGHT FOR THE DAY: *I do experience both hellish and heavenly moments in my life. What if I can go within and just have quiet moments and see what bubbles up from within me over time?*

October 23

---

*"Freedom begins the moment you
realize someone else has been writing your
story and it's time you took the pen from his
hand and started writing it yourself."*
~ Bill Moyers

I seek liberation from a world that tells me who I should be, how my life should look, and what I'm supposed to want. I seek freedom from a culture that tells me what my standard of beauty needs to be, what my body should look like, how much money I need to have, and the careers that make me more valuable. I seek freedom from all the learned limits I was taught to place on myself by a culture that's lost its way.

I am waking up from the murky waters of a world that doesn't praise individuality and works hard to get people to conform. I am waking up to myself, so I get to decide what's best for me. I get to decide how my life should be lived, independent of the cultural beliefs systems that imprison me.

THOUGHT FOR THE DAY: *What if today I can set the intention to awaken even more and see what happens?*

October 24

"I knew that was really the only purpose of life: to be our self, live our truth, and be the love that we are."

~ Anita Moorjani

"Only love it real." This comes from *A Course in Miracles,* and it's a great little mantra to repeat often. The idea behind "only love is real" is that we might see many things that instill fear in us, but below the world view, love is always there. We just can't see it because we're part of a culture deeply embedded in fear.

I want to rip my partner's lips off. Only love is real.

I want to scream at my kids for trashing the carpets I just had cleaned. Only love is real.

I want to pay back my boss for being such a douchebag. Only love is real.

I'm so hurt that my best friend was flirting with my significant other. Only love is real.

I can use this mantra anytime, anywhere. I need not believe it either. Anytime I can tap on what bothers me, that will help, but this powerful little ditty of, "Only love is real," is a very effective pattern interrupt, especially the more consistently I use it. It puts me in touch with the love I am. The love within me.

THOUGHT FOR THE DAY*: What if today, whenever I find I'm disturbed, I can simply say, "Only love is real," and use it as often as needed?*

October 25

"Destroy the idea that you have to be constantly working or grinding in order to be successful. Embrace the concept that rest, recovery, and reflection are essential parts of the progress towards a successful and ultimately happy life. "

~ Manifest Happy

This may be hard to wrap my mind around, but I love this sentiment. I like the idea that rest and recovery from endlessly pursuing one thing after the other is important. Reflecting allows me to go within and allow what needs to come up to surface to do so.

If I lay down my sword of being a constant doer and allow space for life to work through me, rather than me continually pushing, then I find that life can be more fulfilling for me than I thought.

The idea that there is a time to rest, a time to recover, and a time for reflection can be soothing, even if it's not familiar. Allowing myself rest and reflection helps me to act when inspiration is leading the way. As I learn to live in this new rhythm of life, my life unfolds in ways that can amaze me. 🔲SEP

THOUGHT FOR THE DAY: *My life is not meant to be an endless to-do list. What if today I can pause and reflect for 2-3 minutes midday and notice what this does for my well-being?*

October 26

"Before you can hear, much less follow, the voice of your soul, you have to win back your body. You have to go on a pilgrimage beneath the skin."

~ Meggan Watterson

In neuroscience, some say that the body is the subconscious mind. It carries all the unfelt emotions I suppressed. As I learn to unearth and release the suppressed emotions from my body, I learn to love this amazing body. This body is my constant companion through this life. It goes with me everywhere. It carries me through my life and has taken on the incredible task of my unexpressed emotions.

Tapping allows me to release the issues buried in my tissues. This is my way of winning back my body because as I release my suppressed emotions, my body and mind heals. This allows me to connect with my soul, and my pilgrimage beneath my skin has begun.

This is the gift I give to this amazing vehicle that carries me through this human experience.

THOUGHT FOR THE DAY: *My journey beneath my skin is the journey to reconnecting with my soul.*

October 27

"I perceived that I wouldn't have to go out and search for what I was supposed to do- it would unfold before me."

~ Anita Moorjani

The world I live in often talks about finding your purpose and living your dreams. Are my dreams my purpose, then? There's actually a lot of pressure around finding my purpose and living my dreams.

What happens if I never find my purpose?

What if all the dreams I've had don't happen?

How do I feel about myself then? I don't think I feel very good.

What if I could see this whole idea of finding my purpose and living my dreams is a construct of the ego? It has to be, otherwise why would I feel bad if these things don't come into being?

As I learn to determine who's running my show, when I'm feeling bad, it's a clear indication that it's not my authentic self, my higher self in the driver's seat. My authentic self doesn't feel bad. My authentic self is tuned into the truth of my being, and therefore doesn't feel bad about anything. If something isn't working out, this part of me realizes it's not meant to work out because something better is lining up for me. It understands this and allows life to unfold and moves with this unfolding.

There is no searching for what I'm supposed to do. Life may move and work through me rather than me pushing the world's ego-based agenda (like finding my purpose and living my dreams).

This might feel like a huge relief, or it could feel unsettling, or both, but if I go within, I bet I'll find this resonates as true if coming from my authentic self.

THOUGHT FOR THE DAY: *What if I can learn to notice who's running my show and pay more attention to the voice that brings me relief?*

October 28

"If you are falling...dive." ~ Joseph Campbell

I might be scratching my head on this one. What does this mean anyway? It sounds crazy to say when I'm falling, "dive." But what if what Joseph Campbell is suggesting is to release resistance? To actually allow what is to just be, without adding my resistance to the mix? Resistance tends to double down on an already challenging situation. If the thing I resist persists, then maybe Joseph is onto something.

Bryon Katie wrote a book on the topic, called *Loving What Is*. In it she talks about how as I learn to embrace what is, I find peace because I'm in a state of acceptance. If I were meant to be anywhere else, doing anything else, I would be. She's got a point. As resistance to anything—an emotion, a circumstance of any kind—melts away, I will find I move through it easier and thus it moves on easier.

In mindfulness meditation, when I'm experiencing a potent emotion, Jeff Warren teaches the process of hacking whatever emotion I'm feeling by allowing the emotion. To be in a space of non-resistance. If I try this, I can find that the emotion then has the space to do what it's intended to do... move through me.

All of this said, it might be starting to make sense that as I learn to allow what is happening or what I'm feeling to just be, then I'm not in resistance and things have the space to unfold in a way far better than what my resistance brings to the table. I need not believe this, but if I experiment with it, I might find wisdom in non-resistance.

THOUGHT FOR THE DAY: *What if today I can choose an emotion I may not want to feel and practice allowing it to be just what it is, and see what happens with it?*

October 29

"It was then that I understood that my body is only a reflection of my internal state."

~ Anita Moorjani

The body speaks the mind.

The body keeps the score.

The body never lies.

These are all titles of books written on how our emotions affect our bodies. The stress that comes from our emotional state is a powerful force that can affect our physical bodies. Joe Dispenza says, "The body is the subconscious mind." Our bodies reflect our internal state. Anita Moorjani came to see this through her healing crisis.

The world I live in wants to give me a pill or many pills to heal, yet what if there's something deeper that needs to be attended to, to assist my healing. What if disease is a wake-up call for me to go within and see what I might need to attend to in how I'm seeing things in my life? What if a healing crisis reveals this to me? My inner world needs attention. I need to nurture myself and my body more.

The Law of Attraction world tells me that I'm ill because I've attracted it. This feels terrible to tell myself. What if there's a deeper reason I'm experiencing a healing crisis? What if it's awakening me from sleep walking through my life? What if, as I open up to this possibility, my healing crisis is actually guiding me to new perceptions and new ways to live my life far more fulfilling for me?

I like these ideas a lot better than I attracted this due to wrong thinking.

THOUGHT FOR THE DAY: *What if any healing crisis is for my awakening?*

October 30

"When I run after what I think I want, my days are a furnace of stress and anxiety; if I sit in my own place of patience, what I need flows to me, and without pain. From this I understand that what I want also wants me, is looking for me and attracting me. There is a great secret here for anyone who can grasp it." ~ Rumi

This is what the world of the ego teaches—to run after what I think I want. To make it happen. To work hard. To stay focused. To put my big girl or big boy pants on and just do it. This just feels exhausting. It feels stressful and anxiety-producing.

369

I love the idea that if I take a time out and allow things to come, I can find that what I need does comes and without pain and pushing. As Tosha Silver says, "What needs to come can come and what needs to go can go." With ease.

This is a great reminder that whenever I catch myself in working harder, pushing more, trying to manifest, I can pause and ask myself, "Is this the way I'm really meant to live?" and then wait for an answer.

My authentic self resonates with what is light and easy for me. This can be tricky at first because I'm so wired by my culture to push hard, to work hard, to try harder, and to have a plan for my life. In this way, it can feel foreign to me to sit in my own place of patience because patience might not be my strong suit due to the programming.

If it feels uncomfortable, it's just because it's unfamiliar. This can take some time to unhook from. Tapping can help me to move through this so I can get quiet and allow the authentic self to be heard and guidance can come to me for the next step to take.

THOUGHT FOR THE DAY*: What if I'm meant to live in the flow of life rather than pushing hard to make things happen? Just something to consider today.*

October 31

---

*"Fear is normal, expected. But only love
is real."*

~ *Meggan Watterson*

As a human I live in the 3D world that perpetuates fear, anxiety, competition, hard work and so much more. The 3D world pushed the ego's agenda in advertising, many schools, in politics and in the personal development world, just to name a few.

The world's view tells me I need to earn everything. Earn my place in heaven. Earn my success. Earn my worthiness. If I don't fit into this paradigm, or check all the right boxes, then, somehow, I've failed, and I can feel fear. Fear comes from this world.

What if fear is an indicator that something's up? There's something that needs my attention. When I'm feeling fear, there is no space to tune into love, and telling myself that only love is real just doesn't make sense. When I watch the darkness in the 3D world, the idea that only love is real feels farther away than ever.

This is exactly why it's important to interrupt my mind when it becomes too focused on what I'm seeing. What if I can interrupt the fear-filled thoughts, I chip away at programming I keep repeating, and this creates a crack in my beliefs that allow new perceptions to come into my awareness?

I might even find that, over time, I see this 3D world with new eyes, and I experience the truth of what is being said when I repeat, "Only love is real." [P SEP]

THOUGHT FOR THE DAY: *What if it could be true that only love is real?*

November

November 1

"Your success and happiness lie in you."
~ *Helen Keller*

This is the opposite of what the world teaches.

To think that all of this time I may have been endlessly pursuing more of the status that can come in the form of more things.

If I throw in the manifesting world, then it's likely I have been constantly trying to manifest for a long time now. Trying to manifest is exhausting. Pursuing more status or things can feel empty.

This might be a good time to ask myself, "What does success really mean to me, independent of what the world has taught me? What would really bring me a sense of happiness, independent of what the world has taught me?"

I may not know the answers to these questions outside of what I've been told I should want. If I don't know the answers yet, this makes sense because the programming of the world is constant and persistent. What if the answers to these questions come to me as I go within?

If I feel blocked about this, I can tap until I find relief. This opens me up to allow answers to come through me, rather than me "trying," once again, to figure something out. What if I can turn this over to whatever I believe in?

I may have heard that I only need to ask or turn over once and then let it go. I may have also heard that the more I need to ask and turnover, the less

373

likely the answers will come. This presupposes this force for good gets impatient with me and is really no different than a punishing God that has lots of rules I need to follow before any good will be bestowed on me. It's this cosmic asshole who decides who's worthy and who's not.

What if I doubt and ask as often as I need to? What if this force of good is endlessly open to whatever I need to make a deeper connection? I like this version of a Higher Power way better than the punitive one I may have learned.

THOUGHT FOR THE DAY: *What if my sincere desire to connect is all that matters?*

November 2

> *"If the plan doesn't work, change the plan. But never change the goal." ~*
> *Unknown*

This might sound counterintuitive, but if something is not working—if a goal is not coming to fruition—what if the goal needs to be released? And what if it needs to be released because there is something so much better that is lining up to come to me?

If I continue to cling onto a goal, I close myself off from whatever is being lined up to make its way into my experience. I may not trust this idea yet, but doesn't this feel better than telling myself I'm not trying hard enough? That I must not be visualizing properly? Or that I just need to work harder to align myself with my goal?

Triple yuck! It's so much nicer to believe that the force of good has a plan, knows what it's doing, and will guide me to what's for my highest good.

As I release the learned limits I adopted, this opens me up to more synchronistic happenings. My life unfolds in ways even better than my limited self can create goals for, and the goal that didn't work out can be the impetus that connects me in a deeper way to the force of good.

THOUGHT FOR THE DAY: *What if when a goal is not working out, I can consider that it's not meant to because something better for me is coming?*

November 3

"To achieve success then don't doubt your dreams." ~ Ryan D'souza

Oh boy. Here we go again with the nevers. Stick a fork in me, I'm so done. There's got to be a better way.

To tell me to not doubt my dreams... I can see the point, but last time I checked, I'm still human and subject to doubts and fears.

It's far more helpful to remind myself that there's nothing wrong with experiencing doubt and fear. If I stay mired in doubt and fear, then my dreams don't have a chance, even if they're for my highest.

This is where tapping is so helpful in allowing me to attend to my fear and doubt so that I'm not weighed down by them, and I'm not blocking what comes.

If my version of my dreams doesn't come into being, what if it's because there is something that's far better that needs the space to be realized?

In this way, I learn to take steps towards something that inspires me while practicing detaching from a specific outcome. If I become attached, I can tap to help me move back towards freedom.

As I do this, I learn when to step back and wait for guidance and when to take the next step that I'm guided to take. I allow this force of good to work through me. There is freedom in learning to live this way.

THOUGHT FOR THE DAY: *What if I can learn to follow the breadcrumbs that come to me and act when I'm inspired to? I learn when to act and when to rest.*

November 4

> *"Put your heart, mind, and soul into even your smallest acts. This is the secret of success. ~ Swami Sivananda.*

When I act from inspiration, what Swami Sivananda is talking about is easy peasy. When I'm inspired, I don't have to try to put my heart, mind, and soul into my actions. Inherent in inspiration is my heart, mind, and soul being present and accounted for.

This is why it is so amazing to learn to live in a way that's congruent with "doing" when inspiration is leading the way. Otherwise, I'm just another cog in the wheel of life. I might feel important and needed in this role, but I might prefer to be the vehicle that the force of good uses to spread more good into the world.

THOUGHT FOR THE DAY: *What if acting from inspiration is me putting my heart, mind, and soul into whatever actions big or small come?*

November 5

> *"The best revenge is massive success."* ~
> *Frank Sinatra*

This talk of revenge stems from a world that believes in competition. Whenever I compete, I lose. I'm either one up or one down. That's competition. I want to learn to live in a spirit of cooperation. This helps me to see that there's enough room for all of us.

It doesn't matter how many people share my profession, my sense of style, my topic for writing, tapping, meditating, etc. Only I do it the way I do. What if there are people out there right now waiting for what I offer, exactly the way I offer it? This puts an end to this incessant need to agree with the world's idea that there are winners and losers and thus the need to compete to "be the best."

THOUGHT FOR THE DAY: *I'm the best me. I'm unique from anyone else.*

November 6

"There are no limits to what you can accomplish, except the limits you place on your own thinking." ~ Brian Tracy

---

I like releasing learned limits so that I'm open to possibilities I may have thought were impossible for me. What I don't like, however, is this punitive talk that I'm the one blocking myself with my thoughts. Now, it may be true that if I can't see it, I can't create it, but how do I explain the people I have heard about that say they never saw the explosion of good happening in their life coming?

What if they never saw it because they were so focused on each step that got laid out before them? They didn't see it because they were just following the impulses and acting upon them when they felt the urge to? They weren't focused on a specific outcome they were just taking the steps they felt compelled to take. They were following the guidance coming through them. They were detached from the way something needed to turn out.

What if these people were allowing themselves to be used for the highest without being aware that's what they were doing? They were free. What if this can be me, as well?

THOUGHT FOR THE DAY: *What if I can intend to be a channel for the highest to come through me?*

November 7

"Success does not consist in never making mistakes but in never making the same ones a second time." ~ George Bernard Shaw

---

Is this what it takes to succeed? To never make the same mistake more than once? If this is the secret, I think I might be screwed. I can think of more than one occasion where I kept bumping up against my learned limits.

What if each time I bumped up against my learned limits, I was actually slowly but surely waking up to a better way? I just had to exhaust myself from trying so hard so I could wake up from an obsolete way of doing things.

If I go around telling myself that success will only come if I never make the same mistake more than once, I might as well throw in the towel. One can never know the unique journey that each person takes to succeed. This is so true for me.

It's a lot more helpful to tell myself that I can make the same mistake as often as I need to, to awaken. This is part of waking up to a new way of being.

THOUGHT FOR THE DAY: *What if today I can remind myself it's okay to make mistakes and it's okay to make the same mistake multiple times? Each time I do, I get closer to a resolution.*

November 8

---

*"If you want to be successful, find out
what the price is and then pay it." ~ Scott
Adam*

Do I really live in a world where I have to pay a price to have things come to me? Well, in the world of the ego, this is true. This is a world I would like to unhook from. This is a world that leads me to exhaustion, comparison, and more self-judgment.

I'll pass, thank you.

As I learn to allow the force for good to guide me, I need not pay a price. I become the vehicle this force of good uses to spread more good into the world. It doesn't matter if I make a big or a small splash, or any splash in between, because I no longer have to compare myself. I just get to do what comes to me to do and watch what unfolds.

THOUGHT FOR THE DAY: *What if today I can practice acting when I feel the impulse to do so, not because I "have to" or "should"?*

November 9

"Success is a state of mind. If you want success - start thinking of yourself as a success." ~ Dr. Joyce Brothers

---

What if success is overrated when it comes from the world's idea of what success should be? The world tells me I'm successful if I accomplish specific goals. The world tells me I'm successful if I live my true purpose. The world tells me I'm successful by the attainment of popularity or monetary profit. The world tells me I'm successful if I achieve everything I want to achieve.

Do I want these things? It's okay if I do, but I may want to ask myself why I want these things and pay special attention to what follows my "because."

"I want to be successful because…"

My "because" can tell me a lot about myself. My "because" can show me what's operating for me. If I want to be considered a success in this world because I want anything the ego pushes on me, I might want to reconsider my "because."

I might notice the emotions I feel around pursuing the success that the world of the ego pushes. It's highly likely it's not fear or anxiety-free. It's highly likely that this pursuit of success can fill me with fear and anxiety. I can ask myself if there's a way to live my life free of the fear and anxiety that the world pushes on me. This just sounds better.

THOUGHT FOR THE DAY: *What step could I take for myself today free of pushing the ego's agenda?*

November 10

"There is no elevator to success. You have to take the stairs." ~ Unknown

Do I have to take the stairs? If so, I hope it's a stairway to heaven on earth.

I have to take the stairs if I'm following the world agenda. What if there is a better way? What if, as I learn to allow myself to be a vehicle that the force of good uses, things unfold in easy and amazing ways? What if I need not hoof it up the stairs, panting and pushing my way to the top? What if there is an easier way? A happier way, and more fulfilling way?

I like that this could be possible. I like that I could learn to live this way. I like that I can feel more ease, peace, fulfillment and—dare I say it—even happiness in my life. I think I want to rethink this stair climbing prospect.

THOUGHT FOR THE DAY: *What if I can open up to receiving a new way and feel fulfilled along the journey?*

November 11

"Success is no accident. It is hard work, perseverance, learning, studying, sacrifice,

and most of all, love of what you are doing. "
~ Pele

I want to love and be inspired by what I do. This doesn't mean I don't work at it. It means when I take steps from a place of inspiration, the hard work part just melts away. Sacrificing isn't necessary. Perseverance becomes dedication to a better way of living. Learning becomes exciting. Studying is something I aspire to do.

Instead of success being no accident, things work out well for me because I'm no longer "making it happen" or "trying to manifest."

I'm acting from inspiration and the way gets shown and I take those steps. When I do this, amazing things can happen.

THOUGHT FOR THE DAY: *Success is allowing myself to follow inspiration.*

November 12

"Don't just stand there; make
something happen. " ~ Lee Iacocca

This style of personal development is prevalent in this world. It's all about making it happen, and if it's not happening, it's my fault.

Don't just stand there? What if sometimes, it's important to wait? To step back to allow what is being lined up to come in the right time and the right way? Remember the saying, "Whatever the ego creates the ego can lose," By New Thought leader Catherine Ponder.

It might be fair to say that what Lee Iacocca is saying is the voice of the ego, and this is the voice that the world promotes. It's not out of any sinister plan, but rather just because the culture mostly knows no better. Most of us believe this is the way. We are so far removed from the truth of our being that we've fallen asleep to an easier way. A way that's not the ego's creation.

If I follow the slogans that have come from a mostly ego-based culture, I'm more fearful of losing whatever I've gained. If I'm afraid of losing what I've gained, I live in an emotional prison. I'm not free.

If, however, I sit back, allow, and tune into the flow of life—the flow of the force of good—then I live with a lot less fear and trepidation. I'm not in competition with anyone or anything because I know if something doesn't work out, that's because something better is lining up for me. This is a far more peaceful way to live.

THOUGHT FOR THE DAY*: What if there is a time to take inspired action and a time to rest, allow, and wait for the right timing to be revealed?*

November 13

> *"Success happens after you have survived all of your disappointments."* ~
> *Unknown*

There is a lot of truth to this statement.

As I grow weary of the endless cycle of trying to make things happen, I finally stop. I surrender without even knowing it. I'm thinking there's got to be more to life than this endless pursuit of desires and goals. I might have pursued many goals where some came into being and others didn't. Maybe I realize that I'm living other people's ideas of what my life should look like. Any way I look at it, it's not been working well for me. I'm tired of trying so hard with little to no return on what I've been investing my life in.

In this way, it's all the disappointments I've experienced that have led me to this place right now where I want to find a better way. A way that's in line with my soul. The soulful part of me I may have lost touch with a long time ago.

What if these disappointments happened so I could be led back to this place I am now, where my authentic self is calling me back home to myself?

THOUGHT FOR THE DAY: *What if all of my disappointments were leading me back to this moment where I can rekindle this connection to the truest part of me?*

November 14

"No guts. No glory. No legend. No story. —Unknown

How often have I heard statements like this one? Too many to count. If I'm still hooked into the world's view of life, then it's likely that I've beat myself up using statements like this to do it.

Maybe I've told myself that I'm gutless, a wimp, or lacking in the character it takes to be someone bound for glory and bound to be a legend. The bully is running my show if this is the case. And with the bully in the lead, I end up with a story, but it's a sob story about how "I don't have what it takes" and I'll never "make it." What utter nonsense this is.

If I need to throw myself an epic pity party over unrealized dreams, that is 100% okay. I have a right and a need to grieve a loss of what I thought I wanted and the way I thought I should be living. I can use tapping to help me move through my emotions around unrealized dreams. I might find I am open to receiving a new way to see things, and I also might find I do receive a new way of seeing things.

So this, "No guts. No glory. No legend. No story," can now become an entirely new and improved story more about my well-being and connection to my authentic self.

THOUGHT FOR THE DAY*: No more ruts. No more sorry. I'm open to inner glory.*

November 15

> *"For me success is inner peace. That's a good day for me." ~ Denzel Washington*

This is coming from a man most of us would say has reached the pinnacle of success in the worldly way we're taught it. That's how you know you can trust this. Denzel is a mega-movie star. He's an A list actor, a director, and producer. He's got the titles, the status, and that "it" factor. He's a multi-million. He's in a long-standing marriage with a woman he still digs and has four children. He's got this. He can likely check every box on the success list and still he says that success for him is inner peace.

He's been to the show. He's achieved many goals. He's "got it all," and yet he still finds that inner peace is a valuable gauge for success.

Coming from someone who "has it all," he appears to understand what's important and what makes one successful. He's attained what the world tells us to attain, and yet his desire is for inner peace. Now, some might say that because he's achieved this, he has the luxury of desiring more inner peace.

What if, as I learn to tune in to my authentic self, I not only find I feel more inner peace, but I also find that life unfolds for me, so it fills me up? Then I notice I feel abundant. I feel that I'm living a successful version of my life. I'm happy with myself more often than not.

None of this depends on what is in my bank account, my worldly accomplishments (or lack thereof), my relationship status, or how my life looks in any area. I'm content and have more peace than I've ever had before. Then I find I agree with Denzel.

THOUGHT FOR THE DAY: *What if today I can repeat this, "I choose peace in this moment over anything else."*

November 16

"If you don't sacrifice for what you want, what you want becomes the sacrifice."

~ Unknown

Yikes! More talk of sacrificing. Am I meant to sacrifice to have what I want? In the world of the ego, I am.

I want to believe that I need not sacrifice. I want to believe that I need not be tested to see how serious I am about getting what I want. What if, if

I'm needing to sacrifice to receive anything, this indicates that the world of the ego has me firmly in its grip? And what if anything happens that appears as me being tested is actually an opportunity for me to practice more self-acceptance and self-love?

It's an opportunity for me to practice loving myself, especially when I may think I'm not doing it right or getting it right, and I'm filled with self-judgement.

What if I can dispel the idea that I need to ever sacrifice for anything ever again in my life? What if a better way to see this is that what appears to be a sacrifice is actually a redirection to something greater?

THOUGHT FOR THE DAY*: What if sacrifice is a concept of the world of the ego?*

November 17

> *"Never allow waiting to become a habit. Live your dreams and take risks. Life is happening right now."* ~ *wealthygorilla.com*

Haven't I just been learning that waiting is a good thing? Yes, I have. Though I get the point that, as a human, I can be subject to waiting because I'm afraid to act, yet what doesn't get addressed in the world of the ego about this is the fear that's below the surface if I find I'm waiting longer than I feel good about?

What if my non-action is a way I'm unconsciously protecting myself and attempting to keep myself safe? If this feels true, then I can tap so I let go of the need to protect myself in a way that no longer helps me. As I do this, I become open to receiving guidance that becomes easy to act on when the right timing is revealed. No need to push myself to act. I'll just know. I can now act because I'm free of the need to protect myself using waiting to do it.

Taking risks might still feel a little scary when my bully pops in to feed me the worst-case scenario, but I seem to always come back to this sense of knowing I am supported and being directed to what's the highest for me.

THOUGHT FOR THE DAY*: What if waiting is one of two things: it's either the need to protect myself from some fear that might be unconscious, or it's not the right time to act yet?*

389

November 18

---

*"Successful people do what
unsuccessful people are not willing to do.
Don't wish it were easier; wish you were
better." ~ Jim Rohn*

I think I'm seeing a pattern here. These pithy quotes are telling me how success is attained, yet many seem riddled with judgment and competition.

Let me get this straight. I'm an unsuccessful human if I'm not willing to do what these so-called successful people are doing. I'm not successful if I'm tired and worn out from trying so damn hard and yet still nothing has come into being in the way I've been taught it should.

If I'm tired of it all being so damn hard.

I do want things to feel easier, and I want to learn how to live my life true to my authentic self rather than trying to make my life resemble some random construct that got created by a world that propagates the ego.

What if life is actually meant to be way easier than I've been taught? What if I'm not meant to push myself into succeeding in the way the world teaches? What if, as I release more of the learned limits, this feels so much truer? Even if I don't believe it yet, it's worth considering.

THOUGHT FOR THE DAY: *What if easier is the way my life is meant to unfold?*

November 19

"I start early, and I stay late. Day after day, year after year. It took me 17 years and 114 days to become an overnight success. ~ Lional Messi

---

I bet if I went up to any "overnight success" and ask them how they got so successful so quickly, they might laugh and tell me about the lengthy list of things they went through to become an "overnight success", thus dispelling this myth.

What if I can adopt this same attitude towards my connecting with my authentic self? I might not be an overnight success at connecting with this part of me. It might be hit and miss.

Sometimes I might feel deeply connected and tuned in, and other times I might feel lost and discouraged. This is part of melding my humanity with my authentic self. It's a journey that will be ongoing in its deepening. If I know this going on, I can learn to relax about this process. It's a journey I will be on for the rest of this lifetime.

I will have successful connections where I feel in the flow and things seem to magically unfold, and I will have times where I may feel disconnected and hooked back into the world's view, plus every experience between. As I learn to embrace the journey, I will notice that my life flows with more grace and ease when I'm tuned in and not so much when I'm not.

When I have those times where I'm in the flow and following the prompts that come, and act on them, I might chuckle as I think that I, too, am now an "overnight success" in connecting with the force of good that leads my authentic self.

THOUGHT FOR THE DAY*: What if I need not be an overnight success in connecting with my authentic self? What if it's the journey of this lifetime?*

November 20

"Don't tell people your plans. Show them your results." ~ *dreamtime.com*

This is the language of competition. This is the language of the ego (my inner bully). It's haughty and always in comparison mode. It tells me to show others. It sets me against others, and at what cost?

The cost is being in a constant competition with others. When I'm in competition, I lack consciousness. Clients are limited, money is limited, sales are limited, finding a place to live is limited, health is limited, possibilities are limited; virtually everything becomes limited.

I believe in a world where I better rush to get my piece of the pie before someone else beats me to it. My actions become all about getting there first. I might walk over people, betray people, lie to people… the list goes on. This is the world of the ego; it's always filling me with fear, lack, and limitation.

There is no peace in this world because even if I beat someone to the punch and I get there first, there's always the next thing I have to try to get. Manipulation is a big part of the world of the ego.

"It's a dog eat dog world out there." "The world's going to hell in a handbasket."

"Show them your results."

The list goes on.

There's no peace to be found in the world of the ego, and yet peace is what I want. I want more peace and less push. I want more fulfillment and less chasing. I want more cooperation and less competition.

This is why learning to connect with the force of good can bring me such relief. It talks me off the ledge of the world the ego pushes. As I learn to quiet the bully in my brain, I learn to hear the voice of my authentic self. My life becomes far less about "getting mine" and far more about being a vehicle to spread more light into the world. I want more of this, please.

THOUGHT FOR THE DAY*: What if today I can just notice the voice of ego (the inner bully)? Just notice when it's operating. This is a great practice.*

November 21

> *"Not everything that is faced can be changed, but nothing can be changed until it is faced." ~ James Baldwin*

Tapping is a powerful way to face my fears, which are really the learned limits I took on as mine. It can feel daunting to face long held fears and beliefs that have been such a part of me until now, but it is a journey worth taking. The emotional freedom and liberation I gain from doing so make the journey far more palatable.

The years will pass, anyway, so if I'm ready and up for it, the benefits are huge. This said, only I can know if I'm ready for this journey. To push myself before I'm ready is not a good idea, unless this has worked for me in the past with positive outcomes.

I can always start with tapping on whatever resistance I feel about taking this journey without actually diving into the emotional journey. This is actually a great place to see what comes up for me.

The key is to meet myself exactly where I'm at and use tapping to help me see what benefits I get from keeping the status quo in place. As I learn to tap through these, I might find it becomes easier to take the emotional journey because I want the benefits it brings me more than I want to stay the same and not rock the boat.

Only I can know when I'm ready and when the timing is right for me. My place to start is to acknowledge where I stand and tap through that and see what is revealed through the tapping. Tapping works when I use it and when I'm ready. It's all about honoring myself.

THOUGHT FOR THE DAY: *What if today, if I find I'm hesitant to take this journey, I can tap on what's true for me and see where I land?*

November 22

"The difference between successful people and others is how long they spend time feeling sorry for themselves." ~ Barbara Corcoran

Is this really the case? It is in the world of the ego. In the world of emotions, however, it's actually imperative I learn to allow myself my unadulterated truth so I can complete my emotional experience and move on to greener pastures.

This means if I'm feeling sorry for myself, I get to throw myself an epic pity party, provided that I tap my way through it. In this way, I learn to allow the fullness of my emotions to be processed so I don't continue to wallow in feeling sorry for myself.

When I don't give myself this experience, I have pity parties that repeatedly show up and often at inopportune times. This is why telling myself I shouldn't feel whatever I'm feeling backfires and just doesn't work. It actually harms me to tell myself that I shouldn't feel whatever I'm experiencing.

With tapping, I get the full emotional experience, and because of this I find emotional intelligence and freedom on the other side. This continues to grow and expand for me as I continue to allow myself my truth and all the emotions that go with that.

So thank you, Barbara, but I will throw myself an epic pity party while I tap and break free myself from the prison of telling myself I should or shouldn't feel anything.

THOUGHT FOR THE DAY: *Today I begin the journey of honoring myself by allowing myself my full emotional experience.*

November 23

*"Striving for success motivates you.
Striving for perfection is demoralizing."*

~ Harriet Braiker

More striving? I can feel the tiredness weighing down on me. I like allowing whatever is meant for me to come through me a lot better. What if this is me being the most successful person I can be? And what if an awesome life unfolds from this?

I do agree that striving for perfection is exhausting and can end up with me feeling demoralized. I like embracing I am imperfect. I also like letting go of the need to strive for anything.

If I'm striving towards anything, I can ask myself who's voice I'm listening to and then ask myself if this is the voice I want directing my life.

As I continue to wake up from this programming, I will find I want to be kinder to myself and act out of inspiration, not pushing, efforting, or freaking striving. There is a better way, and I mean to live this better way, one day at a time.

THOUGHT FOR THE DAY: *What if I notice whether or not I'm striving instead of thriving?*

November 24

"The goal of life is to make your heartbeat match the beat of the universe, to match your nature with Nature."

~ Joseph Campbell

Wow! This is an alternate reality. What happened to all the talk of succeeding? Is it possible that I do have one big goal in life, and that is to make my heartbeat match the beat of the universe and to match my nature with nature? How might I do this? What would this look like?

What if there is a lot of wisdom here, and what if I need not know the "how" of this? What if the "how" can come to me as I learn how to turn this life over to the care of the force of good? What if this is the truest success in life is to allow the force of good to take over and to be guided and used by the force of good to do its bidding?

Not in a dictatorial way. More of being in the flow that is life. If I look at nature, I can be reminded of how nature doesn't have goals for growth. Birds don't set goals for successful flying, and flowers don't have a plan of action they follow to bloom. They all just are, and they all just allow, and look at how amazingly things turn out.

What if I can learn a lot stepping back out into nature? What if this ignites something in me I need not explain, but I feel renewed? What if I need not try to match my heartbeat to the Universe? What if I can instead practice tuning into my authentic self? What if over time, as I follow the guidance that comes, I notice that my heartbeat is matching the beat of the Universe?

THOUGHT FOR THE DAY: *Within me is a different world waiting for me to tune into it.*

November 25

"The road to success is always under construction." ~ 123rf.com

Okay, I just might love this one. I am always under construction, so why wouldn't my life be as well? I'm learning to create a new, far more personal definition and experience of what success really means.

The more I can learn to embrace I am allowed my own personal definition of success, and the more I continue to unhook myself from the world's agenda for me, the more I find contentment, fulfillment, and inner peace. I might get some push back from family and friends who, like me, have been enculturated to believe in ideas of the ego, but the more I unhook, the less concerned I am about what anyone else thinks about me and my choices.

The interesting thing is as I continue to honor myself, I model for others that they, too, can do the same for themselves, all without saying a word to them.

What can happen is that people stop giving me any push back because I'm so congruent with what I'm doing that they energetically feel this, and they just stop asking.

THOUGHT FOR THE DAY: *I like knowing that I'm allowed to always be under construction.*

November 26

"Success is largely a matter of holding on after others have let go." ~ Unknown

I've likely heard the stories about how successful people keep going, no matter what they face. There is a valiant quality in staying steadfast in what you're doing. I might also agree with this for renewing or beginning a relationship with my authentic self because it is a journey to come back to myself.

The journey back to my authentic self is something that I do daily. It takes practice to learn how to turn my life over to the force of good. It's often counterintuitive to what I've learned. It can seem crazy, even insane to trust that some unseeable force actually has my back. If I practice allowing this force of good to guide my way, the steps begin to be revealed for me to act on.

It may seem crazy because the world is so convincing and so damn loud as to the agenda that it's pushing, so I might feel like I'm insane for even considering a prospect like this. Yet if my life is not working well for me, then maybe it's time to consider another option. What if the world might actually be crazy rather than the other way around?

There is one way to find out. If I experiment with this idea and try it out, I might be pleasantly surprised. On the flip side, I might love turning things over. I trust there is a force for good that has my back and wants what's best for me and knows better than I do. If this is the case, then I can just keep nurturing this relationship.

THOUGHT FOR THE DAY*: What if there is a better way? What if life is so much easier than I've been taught. I need not believe this yet, but what if I can just consider this could be possible?*

November 27

"*A goal without a plan is just a wish.*" ~
Unknown

Is this true? Or could it be possible that I don't actually need goals? I might be thinking, "That's just crazy talk," but is it? And what if I need not plan life or have plans that I'm working on? This might sound like crazy talk.

What if it only sounds crazy because it's something I haven't considered? What if there's never been the space to consider such things because of the way I've been taught? I've been told that I need to set goals and plan to reach those goals and if I don't, I might as well expect to fail.

What if I can tune into a different way to see things? What if so much more is possible that I've ever been able to imagine? This might blow my mind, or it might not.

But if this could be possible, how would I feel about it? How might it change my life? These are things I can contemplate, and eventually I'll know where I land with all of it.

THOUGHT FOR THE DAY: *What if it is possible that I need not set goals and I need not create plans? Just sit with this and let it percolate.*

November 28

"Don't aim for success if you want it;
just do what you love and believe in, and it
will come naturally." ~ David Frost

Does David Frost have information I don't? If I've been on this planet any length of time, it's likely I've heard the ideas that states:

"Do what you love, and the money will follow."

"Follow your bliss."

One is telling me that if I do what I love, I will be taken care of financially. The other statement tells me to just follow what I feel called forward to do from a state of joy, enthusiasm, or bliss.

Joseph Campbell, the famous mythologist, was often quoted as saying, "Follow your bliss and don't be afraid...doors will open where you didn't know they were going to be." This might sound wonderful and scary, but what if Joseph Campbell was tuned into the force of love and knew to say this because of what he came to understand?

It seems like it's good to ponder the idea that if I just follow what makes my heart sing, it will.

What I'm doing as I ponder such concepts is creating a crack in a rock-solid belief system that could use an upgrade.

THOUGHT FOR THE DAY*: What if today I can repeat the quote...in this way...what if it could be possible to follow my bliss and find that doors will open where I didn't know they would be?*

November 29

---

*"We must be willing to let go of the life
we planned so as to have the life that is
waiting for us." ~ Joseph Campbell*

This speaks to letting go of all the plans I have for my life. Letting go of all the goals set to put these plans into play.

This is counterintuitive to what the world teaches, and yet if I've done any contemplating through this book, then I might be opening up to there being a force of good, and this force of good has a plan just for me.

As I release the learned limits the world has placed on me, I learn to let go of how I think life should be. As I do this, I might find there really could be a life waiting for me. What if the force of good is ready, willing, and able to guide me to the life waiting for me?

THOUGHT FOR THE DAY: *What if there is a life waiting for me to live it? A life that's calling me forward.*

November 30

"If something is important enough, even if the odds are against you, you should still do it. ~ Elon Musk

---

This speaks to doing something I feel called forward to do, despite the odds. It also speaks to not putting much weight on how the world sees it. The world could easily poo-poo my idea because the odds are I won't make it.

If I have an impulse to do something and I feel inspired to do so, then it's probably a good idea to act from this inspired place, despite what the statistics or evidence tells me.

What if this is how the force of good speaks? Through the impulses that fill me with inspiration to act.

Allowing this force of good to guide my life opens me up to greater possibilities. I get an idea. I feel strongly about acting on it, despite any naysayers. I may have a sense of knowing I need to act on, and I do. I see what happens, and then another impulse comes, and I feel the inspiration return and I act on that. And on and on.

This is how my life can unfold in amazing ways. This is following the impulses and steps that get laid out for me. This is how I learn to live my life without set goals or set plans.

THOUGHT FOR THE DAY: *What if I don't need goals or a plan for my life? What if there is a force of good that can direct my life so much better than I can?*

December

December 1

"There is a voice that doesn't use words...listen. ~ Rumi

This speaks to when I am acting from inspiration as opposed to the pushing energy of the world. When inspiration strikes it can seem nonsensical, but there's this inner knowing I need to move forward, anyway. A step gets revealed and I take it. Another step gets revealed, and I take the next step. As this unfolds before me, I feel compelled and supported in taking this journey despite the nay-sayers.

Even if fear surfaces, I notice I still feel excited and inspired, and I realize this is part of the journey and I still feel compelled to keep going. If, however, I feel entrenched in fear or debilitated with fear, I can remind myself this comes from me pushing the agenda of the world's shoulds and have to's.

This is the perfect time to step back, regroup, and wait for inspiration to come, and then act once again, but with a different energy. The energy that inspires me, not the energy where I feel like I need to motivate myself to keep going.

It's a learning curve, especially given how entrenched the world is with all the pushing to succeed that it promotes. And it's a journey that has so much more freedom and liberation for me. It's the way it's meant to be.

THOUGHT FOR THE DAY: *What if I can learn to act through inspiration, not desperation?*

December 2

"People say that what we're all seeking is a meaning for life. I don't think that's what we're really seeking. I think that what we're seeking is an experience of being alive, so that our life experiences on the purely physical plane will have resonances with our own innermost being and reality, so that we actually feel the rapture of being alive."

~ *Joseph Campbell,* The Power of Myth

The voice of the world tells me I need to find the meaning of life. This is the ego telling me I need to seek the meaning of life. Yet often my seeking is grasping for meaning. When I'm grasping, things elude me more often than not.

What if I can ask myself, "What would help me to experience being alive right now?" Being in the moment is a simple, yet powerful way to experience being alive. It's a practice.

When I practice just taking a breath, pausing, and taking in what's around me, no matter where I am, or what I have been doing, this is me being in the moment and taking it in. Often, I will notice that the more I do this, the more I genuinely experience being alive. I might also notice that, in doing this, I'm connecting with my innermost being and reality because I'm aware that I'm observing life rather than pushing some agenda that takes me out of the present moment.

As I take more moments like these, this feeling of being alive grows. I find that I'm actually present for my life more and allowing in guidance that moves me forward in joy and fulfillment.

THOUGHT FOR THE DAY: *What if today I can practice being present for 2-3 minutes?*

December 3

"Why worry? What is meant for you is always meant to find you."

~ Indian poet-saint Lalleshwari

Easy to say, harder in practice, especially when I've been wired to worry. Since the ego (the inner bully) is hell-bent on feeding me all the information and evidence as to why things won't work out, to tell myself to simply not worry probably won't land for me. I could feel worse about myself because I do worry. So my worry needs to be attended to. It's also important to let myself off the hook when worry does kick in.

Tapping is a great tool to use (along with mindfulness) to help me interrupt my well entrenched worry pattern. The more I tap or use the mindfulness technique of mental noting (i.e., naming what I'm experiencing in one word, such as "worrying"), the easier it gets to release worry when it's knocking at my door.

By allowing myself my worrisome thoughts and interrupting them, I find they have less of a grip on me and they move on. They might resurface again and again, but my job is to keep interrupting them and then notice how they inhabit my thoughts less and less the more I attend to them. I find that this creates the space for whatever is meant to find me.

THOUGHT FOR THE DAY: *Rather than resist worry or telling myself I shouldn't feel it, I allow it while interrupting it and I find I worry less and trust more, the more I do this.*

December 4

"If you align in any moment with the flow of life as it presents itself, all will unfold in the right way at the right time with a certain spontaneity and ease."

~ Tosha Silver

What a perfect follow-up from yesterday. Another great reminder to practice being in the moment and taking time to do this. As I tune into the moment, I feel the flow of life that presents itself. As I take inspired action steps, the next steps keep getting revealed. I'm learning to allow life to unfold through me rather than me pushing myself towards goals that might not be authentic or true for me. I might wake up to the realization that I've been trying to live someone else's version of a life.

I want to learn to tune into my authentic self and witness the synchronicities being laid out before me. It's such a relief to learn how to allow life to come through me. As I open to the flow of life, I allow in a greater awareness that moves me forward.

THOUGHT FOR THE DAY: *What if I can't be reminded enough there is a better way to live, and this way can be revealed as I learn to allow my authentic self to guide my way?*

December 5

"There are as many atoms in a single molecule of your DNA as there are stars in the typical galaxy. We are, each of us, a little universe." ~ Neil deGrasse Tyson

I know I wasn't taught this. Maybe I was taught I'm limited and that if God gives me good favor because I've behaved appropriately, then I might have a few things I think I want.

Maybe I was taught to reach for the stars while simultaneously being told that I better watch out, and I better not cry, and I better buck up and lead the charge of my life.

Maybe I was taught if things aren't working out for me, then it's my fault and I just need to visualize more clearly or align myself more fully with my desires.

Maybe I was taught something else, but I know that what I was taught about life and myself was not supportive of the idea that I am an amazing little universe all within myself. Whatever I was taught, I would like to awaken to the vastness and beauty of the amazing little universe within me.

There can be many people that might tell me I'm crazy, or blasphemous, or several naysaying (and actually kinda crazy) things. What if this just feels crazy or blasphemous because I was programmed to believe this is so? What if there is another way? A more enlightened and less human way of seeing this life and my place in it? I like that I can open up to this possibility and see what unfolds. Just things to consider.

THOUGHT FOR THE DAY: *What if the Universe does have my back and does guide me? I notice these truths as I unhook from what the world of the ego tells me.*

December 6

"The universe had to fall apart into dust first to become its majestic, incredible, infinite self. What makes you think this breaking, this trauma, this destruction,

won't be the making of a more powerful
you too?" ~ Nikita Gill

Oh wow! So this might mean that it's okay when I fall apart because I have times in my life when I do. As a human on this planet, I do experience breaking, trauma, and destruction.

The personal development world might tell me I need to try harder and do better, but what if the breaking apart is the place where the light comes out from within me? What if this is all part of disconnecting from the world of the ego so I can reconnect with the truest part of my being?

What if anything that I don't like that keeps repeating itself in my life is an opportunity to practice self-acceptance and self-love? What if practicing accepting my broken places, my traumas, and my destruction is part of my journey to true self-love? What if this allows me to receive the goodness intended for me?

THOUGHT FOR THE DAY: *What if self-acceptance of all that I've been through is the key to my freedom?*

December 7

*"The Universe's timing is perfect, even
if it doesn't suit your ego."*

~ Dean Jackson

The Universe's timing doesn't suit my ego because my ego wants me to be prepared for the worst, to stay in fear, to doubt myself.

The ego talks in the language of the bully. It feeds me all the evidence as to why something will not work out, or why I don't have what it takes. It feeds me with fear and doubt about how crazy it is to believe in an invisible force, and especially in a force for good. It makes me wrong every chance it gets, so it can keep me in line and keep the status quo in place.

If I slow down enough to pay attention to what the bully is feeding me, I will see just how crazy this voice is. It leaves no room for possibility or flow and ease. Now that's freaking insane.

I'm sure I can think of something in my life that seemed to unfold for me without me having to push some agenda. This is evidence this invisible force does exist; it has my back, and it guides me to what's best for me.

The more I catch my inner bully (the ego) filling me with fear, the more I wake up from the nightmare it so readily shares with me, and the less I believe the nightmare.

THOUGHT FOR THE DAY: *What if today I can notice when the bully is talking and then simply interrupt it?*

December 8

"Move, but don't move the way fear makes you move."

~ Rumi

Words to live by, and this takes practice. If I keep this as a mantra in my life, I will notice when fear is running my show. When fear is in the driver's seat it gains a lot of momentum if left uninterrupted, and then it has me in its grip with no end in sight.

The bully feeds me a banquet table full of fear every chance it gets. It's often happening within me without my awareness of it. A way to attend to this is to simply set the intention to notice my fear. If I'm so inclined, I can ask for help in noticing when fear is active so I can attend to it.

This soothes my nervous system, which allows better feeling thoughts to make their way up into my psyche. When I soothe my fear, I change the way I see things. I learn to notice the fear, but not allow the fear to be the energy from which I decide.

Fear can still sneak back in and try to take over again, but the more I keep catching it and interrupting it, the less it rules me.

THOUGHT FOR THE DAY: *What if today I can notice, even just once, when fear is trying to get me to move?*

December 9

"God only gives us three answers, "Yes,
not yet, or no, I love you too much"

~ Anonymous

I love the third option.

In the world of the Law of Attraction, the third option doesn't get much airtime. I often hear that if things aren't going the way I want them to, it's because of me. What a wonderful new vantage point to see things from. What a relief. Let me try this on right now and see how this feels.

This thing that I've wanted to happen that hasn't happened yet is my authentic self (or whatever I called it) loving me so much that it's telling me that it's just not the right time, and things are still lining up. What if it's not allowing it so something much better can come to me?

I like it a lot!

THOUGHT FOR THE DAY: *What if when something isn't working out for me, I can remind myself that it's not the right time yet, or that there's something much better being lined up for me?*

December 10

"You are the universe, expressing itself as a human for a little while.

~ Eckhart Tolle

How interesting! This might help me to unhook from the need to find my purpose or to live my dreams. I'm meant to live in a way that's fulfilling for me. The difference is when I think I have to know best, or figure it all out, I can get stuck in the ego's agenda.

What if I can consider that I can be used for the highest? Oprah has often said that her daily prayer is, "Use me for the highest." If I'm the universe, expressing itself as a human for a while, what if this is the perfect prayer or intention to have each day? To allow the Universe to use me for the highest good.

In this way, I need not figure out what my purpose is or how to live my dreams. Instead, I am allowing myself to be a vehicle that the Universe uses. And what if the Universe shows me the how and allows me to feel the flow of life intended for me?

THOUGHT FOR THE DAY*: What if I need not figure this all out?*

415

December 11

"Detachment creates room for creation.

~ Tosha Silver

There is such wisdom in these words. When I grip and try to be in control, I'm effectively cutting myself off from the universal flow. As I learn to release my attachment to how I think things should look, or be, or turn out, I'm allowing in so much more possibility than my ego-based self can imagine. I release the learned limits I learned to place on myself.

I become detached from needing a specific outcome, and I open myself up to the force of good to create through me. I become a vehicle for the highest and best.

Detaching is a process, so when I feel very attached, I can tap, and I can ask for assistance for the universe to free me from my attachment. This is a journey I need not walk alone.

THOUGHT FOR THE DAY: *The Universe creates through me as I learn to let go of my attachments.*

December 12

"If we would just take a moment to look around, we would find that the universe is in constant communication with us." ~ Alexandria Hotmer

---

Mindfulness allows me to tune into the communication always available. It requires my presence to notice. Detachment from specific outcomes creates space for this communication to be heard by me.

This communication can come in a simple thought, or something I hear on the radio, TV, or overhearing a conversation. There is no limit to how the Universe can communicate with me.

What if I can ask for help in hearing the messages? What if I can ask as often as I need to? What if there is no limit to how often I ask for help?

If I haven't been hearing messages for most of my life, it's likely it could take me some time to quiet the voice of the world, so I can hear all the communication always available. There's no shame, ever, in how long I take to hear. My intention to tune in and hear is all that is needed.

THOUGHT FOR THE DAY*: What if I can get quiet for 2-3 minutes and just sit there and do nothing?*

December 13

---

*"Learn how to see. Realize that
everything connects to everything else."*

~ Leonardo DaVinci

I love that Leonardo says <u>learn</u> how to see. It lets me off the hook of needing to know how to see. It's like yoga practice or riding a bike; I learn through practice. I can learn to see the interconnectedness of everything.

What if a great place to start is to consider this idea that everything is connected to everything else? I need not know how or why. I don't even have to believe this. I'm just entertaining the possibility that every person, every experience, every being on this planet, all the stars and planets, the sun and the moon, and all thoughts are, in some way, connected. That's it. Just start here.

It's even better if I allow skepticism and anything else that might surface to come up. I can learn to remove the judgment, over time, about whatever I'm feeling or experiencing. Through allowing any resistance that may come, the judgment just moves along without me attaching to it so strongly. I allow what comes up to come up so it can move and not remain stuck in me.

This is a simple place to start.

THOUGHT FOR THE DAY*: What if today I can contemplate that everything is connected, no exceptions, and just see what surfaces?*

December 14

"...forcing a decision too soon. Often
people intuitively sense what's coming, but
it's not yet time to act. They impatiently try
to push the Flow before God's lined it all
up."

~ *Tosha Silver*

It's highly likely that I've attempted to force decisions. If I have, how has this worked out for me? If I have learned how to step back and allow the needed solutions to come, decisions get made through me rather than me being attached to thinking I know what's best.

Impatience is the voice of the ego taking over.

Pushing results from the ego taking over.

Acting prematurely is the ego taking over.

These can become indicators that I'm allowing fear to move me and choose for me. The fear of missing out (FOMO) is the ego taking over.

I want to learn to see and know when the ego is taking over, so I can attend to this. This allows me to experience the flow of life without all of my ego's meddling.

THOUGHT FOR THE DAY: *I want to practice allowing things to be lined up for me. Awareness of when I'm not is the first step.*

December 15

"Be thankful for what you have; you'll end up having more. If you concentrate on what you don't have, you will never, ever have enough." ~ Oprah

---

Gratitude is such a powerful practice. It's a practice Oprah has made a part of her life for a long time. As I learn to end each day writing down, or just taking in, one thing that I'm grateful for, that's powerful enough to change the way I see things. It can be a very simple thing, like I love the way my cat crawled on my lap and purred.

I love that a cat let me in today.

I love how pretty the birds' songs sounded.

I love that my child smiled at me.

I love that a sweet memory of someone I love came to me.

As I drill down in this simple way, I'm practicing shifting my focus to what's working rather than the litany of what's not working that the bully likes to feed me. Over time, I will notice that I feel better. Even with one simple thing a day, I'm actually training my brain to see what's good. The more I do this, the more good comes because I can see more of it.

THOUGHT FOR THE DAY: *What if today I can start a simple practice of finding one simple thing to be grateful?*

December 16

"To the mind that is still, the whole universe surrenders." ~ Lao Tzu

---

What if Lao Tzu suggests that as I learn to surrender my list of desires, I no longer have to fight my desires? What if instead I choose to be the witness of them? What if my attachment to my desires ceases controlling me?

If I have children or I've been around them, it's likely that if a child is trying to get my attention by acting out and I try to get them to quiet down and sit still, I've likely found they become defiant and actually rebel against my wishes. They may act out in a more animated way.

If, however, I detach from them either by witnessing them with amusement or just ignoring them all together, after enough time passes, the child will lose interest and their energy will diminish. It's not having an effect.

Similarly, when I am fighting against my desires, I give them power over me. If, however, I become the witness of my desires with bemused detachment, this takes away all the fuel that supplies them. Thus, my quietness or stillness actually helps me to release any power they have over me with ease.

This surrendering in me allows the universe to work through me through the power of surrender.

THOUGHT FOR THE DAY: As I learn to surrender to the universal flow in stillness, the Universe can use me for the highest good.

December 17

"Turn your wounds into wisdom "~
Oprah

There is always wisdom in my wounds if I open to this idea. My wounds can be my greatest teacher. It's because of my wounds I may seek assistance, so it brings me back to my authentic self. My wounds are not meant to punish me; they awaken me to deeper truths I might bypass otherwise.

The triggers that come from my wounds are good. They show me the path to my liberation. As I witness my wounds and use tapping to help me release the grip they've had on me, life has a way of unfolding for me that is filled with richness and fulfillment. I've known the dark places, and the lower energies, and now because of these I can feel a greater fullness of life with a lightness of being that has always been a part of me. It's just that now I can feel this lightness with a new appreciation.

THOUGHT FOR THE DAY: What if my wounds carry amazing wisdom in them rather than anything resembling punishment?

December 18

"What you seek is seeking you." ~ Rumi

This Rumi quote encourages me to find a sense of trust and belief that what I am seeking, from my soulful space, is seeking me. This is why I seek it. It is coming through me rather than being created by my ego.

It's the universe letting me know what is intended for my soul's evolution. In time (and with detachment,) it finds its way into my experience at the perfect time and in the perfect way. My only job is to release any attachment to the ego's desires.

It also says that all losses are not really losses because what is meant for me will come, and if it's not meant for me it will go of its own accord. This differs greatly from the idea what I seek isn't coming to me because I'm not properly aligned with it. I like the idea a lot that whatever is meant for me will come, and whatever isn't meant for me will move on.

THOUGHT FOR THE DAY: *What is it for my highest will to come in the perfect time and the perfect way? If it's not meant for me, it will move on.*

December 19

"You were born with wings, why prefer
to crawl through life?" ~ Rumi

The world of the ego clips my wings. It wants it that way. It's fear-based and feeds me a steady stream of everything that can and will go wrong. My upbringing plays a big role in the limits I learned. These limits can come from my parents or other family members, teachers, coaches, religion, or the entire culture I've grown up in.

What all of this programming does is teach me to crawl instead of spreading my wings and fly. I crawl because of the learned limits I've taken on. Another way to say this is that I've put parentheses around my life, and I live within the confines of these parentheses. Throw fear in the mix, and I might crawl even slower throughout my life so as not to rock the boat for those around me who have instilled the limits around my life.

If it doesn't feel safe to fly, I will choose crawling every time. This would answer Rumi's question as to why I might prefer to crawl through life. I'm actually getting a benefit of safety for crawling, and who knows what other benefits I might receive.

Until I learn to release the reasons why it doesn't feel safe to fly, I will continue to crawl. The important thing to know here is that the limits I've been living under have felt known and somehow safer for me. Tapping helps me to uncover the unconscious programming that's in place so I can learn to feel safe while spreading my wings. It's a process, but one so worth it if I find that I'm ready to find my freedom and fly.

THOUGHT FOR THE DAY*: What if today I can ask myself, "What feels safe about things staying the same right now?"*

December 20

"Don't grieve. Anything you lose comes round in another form." ~ Rumi

---

I like the idea a lot that anything that I lose comes back around in some other form, and it's important to allow myself any grief I need to for loss. I need to grieve as a human. I'm still having this human experience, and the emotions that go along with this.

What if it's actually important for me to feel grief when it's in my experience? Telling myself not to grieve when I am grieving is counterproductive. This only suppresses my grief, and it will have to come out somehow at some point.

Allowing myself a fuller expression of grief and tapping through it, when needed, helps me to process my grief and ultimately release it. In this way, I allow myself my human emotional experience, and as I release the grief through feeling it fully, I will find that I'm able to trust that whatever needs to come will come.

THOUGHT FOR THE DAY*: Feeling my grief is important to my well-being. It also allows me to see that whatever is meant for me will find its way to me, no matter what.*

December 21

"The Universe will always remove what is no longer serving you." ~ Gabrielle Bernstein

---

It's interesting to think that if someone or something is still in my life, then it's meant to be there—at least for now. This person or situation may go away eventually, or they may be transformed and appear in a new way. Someone I've struggled with for a long time becomes amiable and easy to be around because I've learned to detach from them and clear out what is within me causing me to be so triggered. I've healed the wound they have revealed.

Whatever needs to leave my life will leave, in the right time and in the right way, as I learn to turn my life and my will over to the care of the Universe. I no longer need to control the situation or the person. I learn to detach from them so there's space for something new to emerge.

I can learn to stop beating myself up because a certain person or circumstance is still in my life and still challenging me. I trust that when my learning is complete, that person will either go away or show up differently.

I trust that when my learning is complete, the circumstance I might have been challenged by clears up because what I needed to evolve is complete.

In this way, I learn to trust the Universe is in charge and knows what it's doing and what is for my highest and best good.

THOUGHT FOR THE DAY: *What if everything is working out for me?*

December 22

"I trust that everything happens for a reason, even if we are not wise enough to see it.

~ Oprah

The view that everything happens for a reason is a nonjudgmental view. The idea that everything that happens in my life is because of how I'm thinking and seeing it places the blame on me.

It makes sense that my attitude has an impact. If I'm consistently thinking the worst, then there's a good bet I will see the worst in situations, and thus believe that things won't work out for me. If I'm consistently seeing the best, then there's a good bet that things will work out for me.

Yet haven't I had experiences in my life that have happened that I gave no attention to? And what about the people who become famous and say they never saw themselves where they're at now?

In these cases, it's not because they've thought themselves into this place. It seems they followed impulses that came to them, and they ended up in a place far beyond where they imagined. Could it be they were following the impulses being left for them to an inspiring end? It would seem so.

When something bad happens to someone, I'll hear that they never in a million years expected this, but they have found value in what they've learned from the experience. What if things happen in my life are meant to help me evolve? I haven't sat around and visualized or affirmed specific things; they just happened. What if they happened because the Universe knows what it's doing and knows how to help me to evolve for the highest good?

THOUGHT FOR THE DAY: *What if things happened through me for the highest good rather than I'm always manifesting or creating everything that happens?*

December 23

"Everything you'll ever need to know is within you; the secrets of the universe are imprinted on the cells of your body." ~ Dan Millman

---

The idea that everything I ever need is within me means any answer I need can come through me as I open up to this idea. I came in with everything already installed in me. There's nothing missing, and nothing I need to bring into me from outside to be whole and free. Over the years, I learned to fall asleep to the truth of my being.

There's a great story about a two-year-old boy who is very persistent with his parents about wanting to be alone with his newborn sibling. The parents finally agree and allow their young son to be alone with their newborn, but they listen on the baby monitor to hear what's happening. What they hear is their son saying to the newborn. "Tell me what God feels like, I'm beginning to forget."

This story has been around a long time, and whether it's a factual event or not, it tells a profound story of how we come in so fresh from God and aware of who we are. Over time and through repetitive programming, we fall asleep to who we are.

Mediation is one way I can practice tuning into my authentic self. My intuitive impulses are the Universe communicating with me. As I get quiet and go within, I can tune into the secrets of the universe imprinted on my cells. I reconnect with my true nature, and all the answers I need can come.

THOUGHT FOR THE DAY: What if everything I need is already within me?

December 24

"The world is full of magical things patiently waiting for our wits to grow sharper."

~ Eden Phillpotts

What if all the things the world sees as magic are the way things are?

Albert Einstein had his views about the world's religions. He believed in what he called "cosmic religion" where God is evident in the order of nature. God's presence is also evident in all aspects and expressions within the universe. Einstein believed that chaos and randomness are not part of nature. Nature moves in an orderly way. Therefore, Einstein was quoted as saying that. "God does not play dice."

There is divine order behind everything. I may have become so far removed from this truth I see chaos and disorder more than the amazing order in it all, yet the Universe never waivers. It just keeps moving forward in this orderly fashion, and as I awaken, I witness that magic is real.

The more I awaken, the more I experience that the synchronicities in life are far more commonplace than I've experienced. My ability to see becomes clearer as I reconnect with the truest part of me. I see that I do live in an orderly universe and I am part of this order.

THOUGHT FOR THE DAY*: What if I can set the intention to be open to see the magic all around me?*

December 25

"Your Source is never a particular person, place, or thing, but God Herself. You never have to beg."

~ Tosha Silver

I live in a world that teaches me that what I need is outside of me, and that I have to do certain things to receive what is mine. I could make a case and show all the evidence as to why my job is my source, or my partner is my source, or I am my source. And yet…

What if my job, myself, and my partner are the vehicles that God uses to bring what is needed into my life? What if the Universe has my back, and as I learn to allow the Universe to take over, things work out well for me? All the pushing and manifesting I've learned that I have to do to create what I want can fall away as more ease and synchronicities unfold before me. I act when I'm guided to and sit back when I'm guided to.

When I remind myself there is a force at work in my life that can line things up far better than I can, I can find relief from the workaholic world I live in. I can find I no longer have to keep going on in the hard way because I experience there is an easier way. The way it's always been intended to be.

THOUGHT FOR THE DAY*: What if God is my source for all, always?*

December 26

"If there is such a thing as spiritual materialism, it is displayed in the urge to possess the mountains rather than to unravel and accept their mysteries." ~ Wojciech Kurtyka

---

In his book, *Cutting Through Spiritual Materialism,* Tibetan meditation master Chögyam Trungpa discusses the most common pitfall to which every person on a spiritual path falls prey to. He calls this pitfall "spiritual materialism." He says, "The problem is that ego can convert anything to its own use, even spirituality."

Spirituality then becomes a process of self-improvement. The tendency is to create a stronger ego by developing and refining the ego. This becomes a never-ending, unfulfilling pursuit to push the ego's agenda and is problematic because the ego is, by nature, essentially empty.

433

Growing up in this world creates this misuse of genuine spirituality because the world pushes the ego's agenda. Genuine spirituality calls me forward to open to a deeper, more profound connection with the force of good. As I practice this, this force moves through me rather than me pushing the agenda of the empty ego with a shopping list of wants.

As Wojciech Kurtyka states, if I'm practicing spiritual materialism, my urge is to possess and manifest more things rather than deepen my connection with the mysteries that surround me. It's helpful for me to witness which I'm practicing, never-ending self-improvement and possession of things, or deepening my connection to the mystery of life that surrounds me.

If I've been practicing spiritual materialism, I find I feel relieved to know a better way enhances my wellbeing.

Thoughts for the Day: What if today I can check in and see what have I been practicing?

December 27

> *"The Universe is saying: 'Allow me to flow through you unrestricted, and you will see the greatest magic you have ever seen.'"* ~
> *Klaus Joehle*

This is the magic that comes from genuine spirituality. If I've been caught up in spiritual materialism, it would make sense because the world I live in pushes this spirituality in every way. As I sink into genuine spiritual connection with the Universe (the force of good), I notice that I do open more to the flow of spirit. I learn to allow myself to be taken over and used for the highest good, As I keep learning to release the learned limits I adopted from the world, the Universe can flow through me unrestricted. As this happens, I witness many things that the world would call magic. Yet what if this has always been the way it's meant to be?

I can learn to tune into the guidance that comes through me so my life can unfold in powerful, peaceful, and fulfilling ways.

THOUGHT FOR THE DAY: *What if I can learn to surrender to the flow of the Universe and allow magic in?*

December 28

"Materialistic way of life is always fearful, because at every step there is danger. Materialistic life is full of anxieties and fear."

~ Srimad Bhagavaram 7.6.5, Srila Prabhupada

What a wake-up call this can be. In the world of spiritual materialism, it says that I am doing well if I am acquiring the things I want. Lifestyle marketing is part of the materialistic way of life. I'm on top if I have the car, the house, the relationship, the career, the money, and the notoriety. It's a seductive world. It's a compelling world. It's a world solidly based on acquiring what the ego's agenda says to acquire.

It's a world filled with comparison and competition. There's never enough of anything for the ego. As soon as I acquire one thing, the next thing appears on the horizon I now need to manifest. My life becomes riddled with fear and anxiety about losing what I have acquired. It turns into an empty and exhausting pursuit.

A deep longing can bubble up inside of me that says, "There's got to be more to life than this." This is often where my journey back to my true self begins. I learn to unhook from the materialistic and the spiritual materialistic world. It's the exhausting journey that brings me to a place where I now seek truth and peace over any one thing.

I step on the path of rekindling a deeper connection to the force of good, and my life feels so much more authentic and true for me.

THOUGHT FOR THE DAY*: What if today I can notice when I'm getting caught up in the cycle of acquiring and just interrupt this pattern, even if just for a moment?*

December 29

> *"Everyone wants to ride with you in the limo, but what you want is someone who will take the bus with you when the limo breaks down." ~ Oprah*

The friends I want are the ones who aren't with me because I provide some status for them. I want friends seeking their most authentic life. A life free of the pursuit of things or needing to ride in a limo to feel that life is good.

Somewhere along the way, the world got wired backwards from the way it's meant to be. I want to be detached from the idea of riding in a limo. In other words, I can take it or leave it. It's not a requirement of any kind. If it happens, that's okay. It might be fun, but it doesn't define me. I want to be detached if I never ride in a limo. I want inner peace and inner freedom more than anything else. If I've been on the gravy train of spiritual materialism until now, I want to get off at the next stop. It may feel uncomfortable for me, but I'll know I'm ready when peace is more important than anything else.

I like that I can learn to release the spiritual materialism from my life so prevalent in our society. I want to learn to march to the beat of my own drum.

THOUGHT FOR THE DAY: *What if today is the beginning of a new way for me?*

437

December 30

---

*"Materialism: Where living beings are
treated as things. Spirituality: Where even
things are treated as spiritual beings."* ~
Glowing Divergence

I want to be the person who treats things as spiritual beings. Maybe I already do, but maybe I'm still grappling with a world that teaches me that my value comes from who I know and what I can show. I want to unhook from a world riddled with the fear and anxiety of more, more, more.

Even spiritual teachers teach that I will always be in pursuit. I am an ever-expanding being, and when I acquire something, it won't be long before the next thing needs to be manifested for my growth and expansion.

I can tell I'm in this cycle by how I feel. If I feel anxious and afraid of losing what I've acquired, then I'm hooked into the material world view, and this view will never bring me peace. I might be fooled into thinking I feel peace, but I'll know it is spiritual materialism because anxiety builds again as I realize I need something new, in a "keeping up with the Jones" fashion.

If I catch this and find I'm making myself wrong for this, I can tap to soothe this self-judgement. How could it be any different given the culture I've been around?

Overtime, I find that my pursuits are far more fulfilling and free of the fear and anxiety that plague me if I'm practicing spiritual materialism. Life flows with more ease and far less angst. The way it's intended to be.

THOUGHT FOR THE DAY*: What if today I can tune in and notice when I'm feeling pressure and fear and tap to find relief from this?*

December 31

"The main point of any spiritual practice is to step out of the bureaucracy of ego. This means stepping out of ego's constant desire for a higher, more spiritual, more transcendental version of knowledge, religion, virtue, judgment, comfort, or whatever it is that the particular ego is seeking. One must step out of spiritual materialism." ~ Chögyam Trungpa

This is a great way to end this year. If I've been in pursuit of new and improved spiritual practices or experiences, I can awaken to the realization this is the ego pushing its spiritually disguised agenda. It's the wolf mask in a spiritual sheep's clothing. It's the super sneaky way the ego (the inner bully) communicates with me. It can sound like this…

"You need to go to that retreat so that you can become more enlightened."

"You need to create a spiritual program to help people wake up from their ego."

"You need to create a new vision board and meditate on it daily."

"You need to go deeper into visualizing what you want, so that you can manifest it."

"If you're not manifesting what you want, you're in resistance."

"If you follow my 5-step program to manifesting your dreams, you'll manifest your dreams."

I've seen and heard a thousand quotes that sound good on some level, but how do I feel when I don't manifest what I think I should want? I don't feel good. I go to self-judgement and self-blame. These are indicators that the ego has me by the short-hairs, and it's a good time to interrupt the madness of the ego so I can eventually hear what the force of good is guiding me to.

I step away from the world of the ego and all of its empty pursuits, and I wake-up to the guidance always there for me. It's just required some interrupting of thought patterns with a lot of momentum. The more consistently I tap to interrupt these limiting thoughts, the better I feel. I learn to surrender to the Universe that knows what's for the highest and has my back, and my life gets better and better.

THOUGHT FOR THE DAY: *I prefer peace over anything.*

About the Authors

Marti Murphy is an Emotional Fitness Coach, a Certified EFT Practitioner, and Psychosomatics Practitioner, Marti is a life-long self-improvement junkie who was always on the hunt for peace and happiness. But it eluded her. She tried positive thinking, but it never stuck for long. This book walks you thought simple suggestions to help allow positivity in naturally.

Bailey Samples graduated from Colorado State University with a Bachelor of Science in Psychology. She's a major contributor to this book project and to the original book—*Forbidden Emotions: The Key to Healing*— as an editor and co-writer. She works at The Institute for Conflict Management based in Seattle Washington.

About JEBWizard Publishing

JEBWizard Publishing offers a hybrid approach to publishing. By taking a vested interest in the success of your book, we put our reputation on the line to create and market a quality publication. We offer a customized solution based on your individual project needs.

Our catalog of authors spans the spectrum of fiction, non-fiction, Young Adult, True Crime, Self-help, and Children's books.

Contact us for submission guidelines at

https://www.jebwizardpublishing.com

Info@jebwizardpublishing.com

Or in writing at

JEBWizard Publishing

37 Park Forest Rd.

Cranston, RI 02920